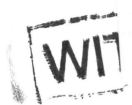 

Being Me and Also Us

Lessons from the Peckham Experiment

Alison Stallibrass

Scottish Academic Press

© Alison Stallibrass 1989
Introduction © Leila Berg 1989

First published 1989

Scottish Academic Press
33 Montgomery Street
Edinburgh EH7 5JX

British Library Cataloguing in Publication Data available

ISBN 0 7073 0599 3

Printed and bound in Great Britain by Billing and Sons Ltd, Worcester
Designed and typeset by Fine Line Publishing Services, Witney, Oxon

To the Peckham Biologists

Acknowledgements

I would like to express my very sincere gratitude to former members of the staff of the Pioneer Health Centre and other friends who have read and criticised – often in very healpful detail – drafts of the book at various stages; in particular, Rosemary Frost, Mary Langman, Allan Pepper, Dr Kenneth Barlow, Dr Robert Bolton, Rabbi Rachel Montagu, Dr Geoffrey Richman, Marie Richman, Elsie Purser, Celia Eatwell, Geoffrey Stallibrass and William Stallibrass, and to Leila Berg who encouraged me to attempt this book and contributed the introduction. I would also like to thank the former members of the Centre who have helped by searching their memories and telling me their recollections. Their names appear mainly in chapter 7.

The excerpts from *Holism and Evolution* by Jan Christian Smuts are reprinted by permission of A P Watt Ltd on behalf of The Society to Help Civilian Blind.

The excerpt from *Studying Children* by Ross Vasta is reprinted by permission of Ross Vasta.

The excerpts from *Origin of Intelligence in the Child* by Jean Piaget are reprinted by permission of Routledge and Kegan Paul.

The excerpt from *The Growth of Competence* by J Bruner and K Connolly is reprinted by permission of Academic Press (Orlando).

The excerpts from *The Continuum Concept* by Jean Liedloff are reprinted by permission of Jean Liedloff.

The excerpts from *Politics and History in Band Societies* by Richard Lee and Eleanor Leacock are reprinted by permission of Cambridge University Press.

The excerpts from *Gaia: a new look at life on earth* by J E Lovelock are reprinted by permission of Oxford University Press.

The excerpt from *Pattern and Growth in Personality* by Gordon W Allport is reprinted by permission of Robert Allport.

The excerpts from *Beast and Man* by Mary Midgley are reprinted by permission of Methuen and Co Ltd.

The excerpts from the work of Stephen Boyden are reprinted by permission of Stephen Boyden.

The excerpt from 'Tumble Tots' in *Nursery World* is reprinted by permission of Nursery World.

Introduction

Axolotls are dull, stupid animals. They look like enormous tadpoles, six inches long. People used to keep them in tanks in their sitting rooms. There the axolotls blundered about, not looking, not caring, not even wondering.

Yet because they grew up, had children and grew old, people said, 'Well, that's how axolotls are and always will be.'

Salamanders are quite different. They are lively lizards, who love sun and light. They see clearly where they are going, and run wherever they please, relishing life.

One day a scientist discovered that if an axolotl is given the right food and right kind of help, it changes and turns into what it was always meant to be – a SALAMANDER!

This is printed at the beginning of a series for young children I edited in the early sixties, a series I even called *Salamanders*.

I had read years before in *The Peckham Experiment* that because axolotls had lived out in their sluggishness a complete life cycle, no-one, including zoologists, had ever suspected the actual truth, which was that they were an uncompleted form of a very different animal.

This was an amazing revelation that affected my whole life. I think the Peckham Centre took many people that way. It was something blazingly new, yet at the same time something you had always known, so that you felt you had simultaneously both shot to the stars, and come home.

That is why it is so difficult to write about the Centre *briefly*, as I have been asked to do. Just as it drew in so many people – cleaners, lawyers, dustmen, artists – it also touched on so many aspects of life – education, medicine, philosophy, architecture. I don't think we had the word 'holistic' then.

I can pick up *Look at Kids* and read what I wrote years ago about an intelligent four-year-old I played dominoes with: how when my dominoes fell over so that he could see them, he studied them intently – and then chose from his own pile not one that would beat me, but one that would keep the game going.

He did it not because he was altruistic, or self-sacrificing, but because he needed the game to continue, he wanted our relationship – our co-operation – to continue. To win – that is, to destroy the pleasant relationship-in-existence – was an idea quite alien to him. But an authoritarian adult would have taught him to win – and to destroy what was important to him, and ultimately to believe that winning was what he wanted.

Of course I had imbibed that way of looking from reading about the Peckham Centre.

When I wrote about finding myself in a crowded London Underground passage, dodging to the right, to the left, to try to get round a similarly frantic man in front of me who mirrored my movements, I was remembering the small children in the Centre nursery gym, not trying anxiously and egotistically to avoid each other, but swinging and moving intuitively into space, seeing the total situation.

And when I started to run a writing-for-pleasure group for over-60s where I now live (because several people wanted to have such a group and asked for someone to run it) I said it would not be a school or a college that taught rules and made judgements, because I unconsciously remembered that Dr Scott Williamson and Dr Innes Pearse had said that in the first year and a half of the Centre they learned that all people, from infants to old, resent being instructed. 'The voice of the teacher,' they said, 'frightens the potential users'; and impatience, even when it's called helpfulness rather than compulsion, strangles creativity. The Peckham voice has worked well for us.

A few days ago I was in a London bus, seated between two elderly women, strangers to me, talking across me. 'Going to Bingo, are you?' 'Yes. Go every afternoon. Can't sit staring at your four walls all day, can you? Go bleeding mad!' And she got off outside the hall, having made it clear that she didn't *choose* Bingo - except as an alternative to going mad from isolation. Yet the old-age pensioner, a woman generally, who goes off daily to Bingo, is patronisingly or scornfully accepted as a normal part of our present society. The next day I was among a dozen people age 30 to 70-plus, watching a video about non-professional helpers looking after people who were dying. We had a very lively and long discussion afterwards, which began to settle somehow on old people's homes, where 'inmates' sat silently slumped in chairs. I spoke of the women I'd sat between on the London bus. 'You need children running about,' said someone. 'People of all ages.' 'A sort of club,' said someone else. 'Why don't we have something like that?' 'We did once,' I said. And I started to tell them about the Peckham Centre. And as we picked up coats to go, they began to say, 'We should start one again' and 'What would we call it?' And not with any idea of answering this question, but just to give a last bit of information before we separated, I told them about the axolotls. 'That's it!' said one. 'We'd call it Salamanders.'

Leila Berg

Contents

Prologue

This book describes a social experiment of fifty years ago, famous in its time but now only hazily remembered, that urgently needs to be recalled and understood. For there is a chance that the knowledge of human needs and possibilities that was gained from it could, if widely absorbed and applied, improve the overall capability of human beings to deal with the avalanche of social, economic and ecological problems that threatens to destroy mankind.

What is this knowledge for which so much is claimed? First, what it is not. It has nothing to do with genetic engineering. It is neither a political nor an economic programme, nor a series of moral precepts to be followed. It does not tell us how to cure the sick, support the incapable, direct the young or force or cajole people into any mould; it is not in any way a knowledge of what one might try to do *to* people in order to improve them.

What was gained through the experimental Pioneer Health Centre, better known as the Peckham Experiment, was knowledge of the basic nature and needs of human beings.

The directors of the experiment wanted to study healthy people, and in order to do that they had to find out how to create circumstances in which people are able to cultivate physical, mental and emotional health in themselves.

This account of the experiment and of the insights that inspired it and were confirmed by it will, I believe, be welcomed by the many people who are trying to create the physical and social conditions around them in which they and their children may develop their potentiality for skills, wisdom, joy-in-life and love, in continuing and creative association with their neighbours. For people are feeling a lack of community life. There is a growing awareness of the fact that just as a child needs to feel that it is an active part of a social whole – a family or a small stable group – in order to gain, among other things, a sense of identity and worth, so a family needs to be a creative part of a greater social whole – a neighbourhood community, if it is to be healthy and to serve a useful purpose.

Today, the climate of opinion is altogether much more favourable to the understanding of the Peckham Biologists' vision of health and of the conclusions they drew from the results of their experiment than ever it was before. There is a growing awareness that the opportunity to become, in childhood, both capable of and desirous of directing one's own life, of thinking, feeling and choosing for oneself is essential to the health of individuals and of the society they create. People are looking for answers to such questions as, 'What sort of opportunities for action and interaction do human beings need, if they are to be able to develop their potential capability?' or, 'What sort of conditions of life will foster real and lasting freedom, individuality, responsibility and creativity?'

Much may be learned about the basic physical and social needs of humankind from an open-minded study of the lifestyles of peoples who have lived in a rational and mutually beneficial relationship with nature, during and since prehistoric times – while civilisations have come and gone. Since these predominantly 'hunting and gathering' peoples have now been squeezed into the most inhospitable corners of the Earth, and if having succeeded in maintaining, in spite of this, a healthy way of life, may not want to divulge their hiding places, we have to rely almost entirely on the reports that have already been published by professional and amateur anthropologists. These are fascinating.

Another welcome development has been the work of animal etholo-gists. Students of animal behaviour are spending years of their lives watching, describing – and filming – the behaviour of animals, birds, insects and fishes in the wild. People are able to witness on the tele-vision screen the most astonishing and wonder-arousing phenomena, such as the parental care of crocodiles. This is perhaps increasing our respect for nature and our fellow living beings. One of the things we may be learning is that a particular species needs a particular kind of environment if it is to flourish, or, rather, that there is a limit to a living creature's power to cope successfully with changes in its environment. Perhaps this will stimulate us to wonder what kind of an environment human beings need from birth to old age, if they are to be happy, healthy and wise. The Nobel prizewinner, Niko Tinbergen has said:

> We are creating a habitat that diverges more and more and with increasing speed from that to which genetic evolution has adapted us.[*]

He urges 'a restoration of a tolerable environment and the development in ourselves of the highest possible level of flexibility', and passionately calls on 'all sciences concerned with the biology of man to work for an integration of their many and diverse approaches, and to step up the pace of the building of a coherent, comprehensive science of man.'[†]

And time is short. We cannot afford to neglect the work that has already been done. Together with the knowledge that is fast accumulating of the nutritional needs of the body, the Peckham Biologists' theoretical and experimental work on the nutritional needs of the soul – or whatever the rest of the human organism may best be called – could fill to a large

[*] The Croonian Lecture 1972
[†] *ibid.*

extent this tragic gap in the knowledge and wisdom of our world-wide civilisation.

I hope this book will help to make their insights and discoveries available to students of the 'Life Sciences', and to all of us, we the general public, from whom the driving force for change in our priorities and values must come.

The science of psychology has concerned itself mainly with the study of the sick and of how to heal them. Its theories of how humans function have grown out of this work, but, during the 1950s, some psychologists saw the need to study healthy subjects and to discover the nature of healthy human nature, to create a psychology of health. This 'school' or, rather, loose association of original minds has been called 'The Third Force' to distinguish it from the existing two main 'schools', the psychoanalytical and the behaviourist. It is also referred to as Growth Psychology, and is associated with Abraham Maslow, Carl Rogers and Gordon Allport among others. Maslow made a series of studies of people who did not appear to be suffering from any symptoms of psychological ill-health, were also capable and self-directing and who seemed to have made the most of their innate capacity and their environmental circumstances. He came to the conclusion that they could best be defined as 'self-actualising' or fully human people, and he described them also as 'efficiently perceptive', 'spontaneous', 'autonomous', 'caring' and 'responsible'. Some of Maslow's subjects for study were public figures or exceptionally circumstanced, but in the conditions obtaining in the Peckham Experiment, numbers of people with ordinary backgrounds and occupations could be described in exactly that way. I am amazed at how well the adjectives used by Maslow (as quoted above) to describe the individuals he considered to be healthy fit my memory of the men, women and especially the children who had been enthusiastically taking part in the experiment for a year or two.

When I say taking part, I do not mean in the least that they consciously sought self-improvement. What happened was that they joined the club out of curiosity, because they were lonely, or for a variety of other reasons, and found that it provided them with the circumstances in which they were able to function in a way that promoted their health and happiness. For them, the Peckham Pioneer Health Centre was a family club which became the centre of their social lives and an extension of their homes. They and the staff referred to it simply as 'the Centre'; to George Scott Williamson MC MD and Innes Hope Pearse MD, it was, they said, 'their laboratory'. It was the means whereby they hoped to learn about health and about the kind of environmental circumstances that enable people to cultivate health in themselves and their children.

When Williamson and Pearse used the word 'health', they meant health; they did not use it, as is usual today, as a synonym for sickness as in 'health service', 'health authorities' and 'health centres' (group practice surgeries), or as meaning 'therapy' as so often in the phrase 'holistic health'. Nor did they mean merely a state of being free from pain and able to carry on after a fashion with one's daily tasks. Health to them meant vitality, joy in being alive and in the life around one; it meant ease and order in bodies and in social bodies in contrast to disease and disorder; it meant the full development of a person's human faculties and individual talents. Not that health is easy to recognise because it does not call attention to itself; its characteristic manifestations are 'so natural, so easy that they go unnoticed'.*

In *Biologists in Search of Material* (1938) they wrote:

> Man's vaunted conquest of nature is the expression of a power complex
> – vain humbug. Nature is that which we obey... We must strengthen our
> humility to hasten the era of greater obedience.

In the 1990s, far more than when it was written, this will strike home. There is a growing awareness that we are a part of the natural world and, potentially, as wonderful as any other living creatures, and that we are not gods, free to do as the fancy takes us, nor are our children machines that we can fashion as we please. The uncomfortable thought begins to obtrude that our future as a species is at risk because of the way in which we behave. For example, people are beginning to realise with horror that much of the food and drink on sale to the public contains materials that no human body can tolerate for long. More than forty years ago, Scott Williamson and Innes Pearse were already aware of the need to find out about the biological laws governing the nutritional needs of humans and the health of the soil and water in which food is grown; they were founder-members of the Soil Association†. But their particular gift to posterity was the conception – and the practical confirmation in their 'laboratory' – of a theory of the nature of the biological laws that govern the full and healthy development of the humanity and individuality of human beings, and the kind of physical and social circumstances in which these laws can freely operate.

The fascinating reports of their work by the directors of the experiment and their senior colleagues are still in print; I hope this book will act as an introduction to them. I want to make it clear at the outset that it is not intended to be a definitive history of the experiment; nor is it likely to contain a complete account of the founders' answer to the question they asked – what is health and how is it to be acquired – but only so much of it as I have been capable of understanding and making my own. It contains my personal interpretation of their theory and practice as well as my memories of the Centre and those of some former members and staff. However ill-equipped I may be for the task I have undertaken, I should never forgive myself if I did not attempt it. It is

---

* 1965, Author's Note
† The oldest of the organisations devoted to research into soil health and organic farming.

also my delight to do so. I am for ever grateful for having had the opportunity, as a young woman, to spend three years soaking up experiences of the Centre and listening to informal discussions between the two directors and their colleagues, while I was acting as a student-assistant to Lucy H Crocker, in that part of her work which consisted in providing play opportunities for the children of member-families. During these three years, I felt that I was assisting in an enterprise that offered the best chance there was of changing the world for the better. The memory of it remained at the back of my mind; and, all the while I was bringing up five children and running, for fourteen years, a pre-school playgroup (where I tried to treat the children as we had treated the Centre children), I believe I was digesting the experiences and ideas I had encountered at the Pioneer Health Centre. During the last twenty years, while looking at theories of child development in the light of recollections of the behaviour of the children in the Centre and in my playgroup, and writing on the subject, my understanding of the Peckham Biologists' theory and practice has clarified and I feel capable of putting it into words.

Long-term members of the Centre felt passionately its rightness and value for themselves and their children. To hear them speak of it today, after the passage of thirty or more years, leaves one in no doubt of that. The action they took in 1946 and again in 1950 is evidence of the fact. Four and a half years after its opening in May 1935, the outbreak of the Second World War forced the Centre to close. (It was considered to be too danger-ous for large numbers of people to be congregated near the London docks in a building largely made of glass.) But, immediately hostilities ceased, families who had been members and still lived in the area or nearby mobilised themselves to get it reopened. They met in each others' homes and then in church halls and finally hired a large hall and called a meeting, which was attended by well over 1,000 people, and invited Doctors Wil-liamson and Pearse to speak. Many offered their time and skills to clean and repair and refurnish the building, which had been used as a munitions factory, and implored 'the Doctors' to find some staff and money. They also offered to pay double the pre-war family subscription. When the Sir Halley Stewart Trust offered a grant of £10,000 a year for three years, on condition that the Centre was reopened immediately, it was decided to do so in spite of the difficulties caused by wartime shortages and the fact that most of the pre-war staff were no longer available and all the equipment had been given to the war effort. Housing was bad in the area due to the age of the buildings, bombing and neglect, yet, of the 875 families that had been fully paid up members on the outbreak of war, 550 rejoined at once. They set to and repaired and cleaned the building which was covered with machine oil and the grime of years. They held a memorable opening party to which 3,000 people came and, the next day, the building was humming with activity just as if there had been no break of seven years. It was observed that these families seemed to know, more clearly than ever before, exactly what they wanted of their Centre.

Four and a half years after reopening, it came to an end for lack of funds. The reasons for the financial failure are discussed in a later chapter. When they heard that the Centre was bankrupt and would be forced to close, the members were dumbfounded. Their confident hope that their children would be able to grow up enjoying the community life, the fellowship, and the health and confidence that membership of the Centre gave was shattered. Many were moved to press for support in high places. Some of these, who have been asked to recall those days, say they are astonished to remember the courage with which they, as representatives of the membership, penetrated the House of Commons, where they tried to interest a gathering of women Members of Parliament and, later, a group of the Labour Members of Parliament for the London Boroughs, and also the headquarters of the London County Council where they argued their case for hours on more than one occasion – all to no avail. One of the many letters received by the two Doctors at this time began:

> With the Centre as my background, there isn't anything I would not tackle. It has given me such confidence, a thing I never had before. When I realise that my children are having that background from the beginning, I know what a much fuller life they will lead. The Centre is something they cannot do without.

and ended:

> Summing up from us all, I would say that we have been given something by belonging to the Centre which, should it close, will never be taken away. With gratitude we all thank you for this.

Part One

The Story of the Experiment

Chapter 1

A Pilot Scheme

In the mid-1920s, a small circle of friends (mostly youthful married couples, some with money at their disposal) were united in feeling strongly that the benefits of information concerning effective and hygienic methods of birth control should not be the prerogative of the rich. They set themselves the task of finding a means of extending these benefits to all despite existing laws.

It came to their knowledge that during her seven year long stint of work at the Alice Model Infant Welfare Centre in Stepney, Dr Innes Pearse had repeatedly expressed her conviction, in her annual reports, that it was impossible for the women attending the clinic to rear healthy children unless they were able to space their pregnancies more widely. At this time, Dr Pearse was assisting George Scott Williamson in his research into the structure and function of the thyroid gland at the Royal Free Hospital. One day, Dorrit Schlesinger, representing the group of young philanthropists, called to see Dr Pearse in the pathology department of the hospital.

The two women had been conversing animatedly for a little while, when Mrs Schlesinger heard the noise of a chair scraping on the floor and a man emerged from within a large black bag, suspended from the ceiling in a dark corner of the room, which served as a photographic lab, and introduced himself as George Scott Williamson. He said that, in his opinion, decisions regarding the use of contraceptives were for wife and husband to take together as a part of their mutual regulation of their family life. He believed it important that information on the control of conception should be given to the man and the woman together and that they should have the opportunity to discuss the question with the medical practitioner, and thus be able to take a better informed responsibility for the health and happiness of the family as a whole.

Innes Pearse was equally certain of the uselessness of a piecemeal technique of 'welfare'. At the infant welfare clinic, she had been almost unbearably frustrated by the fact that she was not allowed to examine the mother, who often looked so tired and ill, and advise or treat her. The fathers she never saw.

Mrs Schlesinger was impressed. She arranged a meeting with the rest of the group, who decided that Scott Williamson and Innes Pearse would be preferable to another medical expert that they had had in mind for the project. Before long, the two doctors had infected the group with their enthusiasm for the need to discover how to enable people to be effectively responsible for their own and their families' health (in the unadulterated sense of the word) and how to enable the medical practitioner with his specialist knowledge and skill to assist them most effectively to do so.

In their intention to make information on birth control more widely available, the group were motivated by the desire that families should be happy. They reasoned that unhealthy children are not happy; therefore, they shared the Doctors' interest in studying how to promote health. They felt, above all else, that the parents should want the child but also that they should be as capable as possible of giving it a healthy start in life. So they must be as fit as possible when the child is conceived and carried, and have access to up-to-date knowledge of how to provide children with as healthy an environment as their circumstances might permit.

The group decided to set up an experiment in order to find out if people would welcome the opportunity to obtain information regarding the state of their physical fitness and would also like to be helped to assume the responsibility for their own health and that of their children. They formed a committee which loyally supported Scott Williamson and Innes Pearse in their research into the nature of health for as long as the work lasted. One of the original members, the Hon Mrs Ewen Montagu (Hon Sec for 40 years), is still serving on the executive committee of the Pioneer Health Centre Ltd which survives to keep the memory of the Centre alive and to encourage any similar projects.

A word now on the two doctors' backgrounds: Innes Hope Pearse (1890–1979) was the only child of well-to-do parents and had a very lonely childhood. What saved her, she said, was being turned out every day into the large enclosed garden. There she could roam at will, 'climb trees, play with the rabbit and get to know every insect that crawled in the grass ... the gardener was friendly, but the cook was horrible'. Her parents seem to have been merely remote. Later she was sent to a school in Croydon and made lifelong friends, but she suffered from shyness all her life; this was hidden by her colourful personality and downright manner. She loved art, crafts and dress designing but chose to study medicine because she felt it was a career that would give her the freedom and effectiveness she craved. Her fellow students called her 'Peter Rabbit' – Pete for short, and Pete was the name she adopted and kept for the rest of her long life.

She qualified at the Royal Free Hospital in 1916 and after working at the Bristol Royal Hospital for Children and Women and the Great Northern Hospital, she applied in 1919 for a house appointment at the London Hospital. She was told, 'We don't have women here.' But she persisted;

she knew that the war had caused a shortage of doctors. Eventually they said, 'Yes, if you can bring three other women.' This she was easily able to do, and she became the first woman medical registrar at the London Hospital. Later she held the post of surgical registrar at the Royal Free Hospital. There she met Scott Williamson and, her ambition to make a career as a surgeon having been frustrated by a severe illness, she became his assistant in his teaching work in the hospital and the research he was doing on the structure and function of the thyroid gland.

George Scott Williamson (1885–1953) was the eldest child of a Newcastle sea captain and his Scottish wife. Of the seven children, five boys and two girls, four became doctors of medicine. He had a very great admiration and affection for his mother to whom, because of the absence of her husband at sea, fell the task of bringing up the children. When twins were born, he used to hurry home from school in order to help her with their evening bath before the fire, enjoying the opportunity for a quiet chat with her.

His writings show a respect for feminine wisdom. He observed that women and girls – even little ones – are, in general, more interested in and concerned with people and other living things – things that grow – than in objects and machines, abstract ideas and the artificial putting together of things which is, on the whole, the male tendency. It seemed to him that this female bias can give women a greater realism, can keep their feet firmly on the ground and their ears closer to the secrets of nature and the fundamental needs of humanity.

> I was thirteen when a small sister died of 'broncho-pneumonia'. A brother of five, to me a very 'special' brother, also lay desperately ill. I used to sit on his bed wondering what I could do to ease his breathing. I kept putting my finger down his throat and pulling out the phlegm that seemed to be choking him. He recovered. It was only much later, when I was grown up, that I knew it was diptheria they had both had. I then began to ponder how I had escaped; for I had actually been handling the deadly membrane: and I don't suppose I had even washed my hands with any special care! So I came to realise that a so-called pathological 'cause' is not necessarily followed by a pathological 'effect'. Was there, then, some intrinsic process of health working alongside, but distinct from, the well-established sequential process of disease?*

He later wrote:

> In 1899 when I was sixteen I had a rash – 'scarlet fever' – and I was carried off to the fever hospital. Two days later it was decided that I had not got scarlet fever: but I was kept in the hospital a further fortnight in case I took the fever in the hospital. I spent my time helping the nurses – for that was a long time ago.
>
> But why did I not get scarlet fever when I had actually been in a scarlet fever ward? The same question again: there must be a positive

* *The Quality of Life* (Appendix no. 1)

process of health as well as, and different from, the process of disease. I decided I must find out. So I became a doctor.*

In 1903, when he was a medical student in Edinburgh, there was an outbreak of smallpox. He volunteered to help on the smallpox isolation ship. He wrote:

> The first case I saw was a woman dying of malignant smallpox. She was at full term, but was past all hope of recovery or of delivering the baby. The superintendent, deciding that it might just be possible to save the baby, did a Caesarean section. From the body of the dying woman, black with lesions of smallpox, was taken a perfect shell-pink infant. Health again! – in the midst of deadly disease.[†]

His thoughts returned often to the mystery of natural immunity and insusceptibility. 'Why', he wrote, 'were some people able to live in harmony with what to others was a deadly insult?' He decided that the study of the pathological processes underlying disease might enable him to solve the mystery. So he specialised in pathology.

Later he wrote:

> As a university lecturer in pathology, I spent some time helping a friend who was experimenting with the infectivity of airborne bacilli. I made the emulsion of live bacilli and this we puffed freely into the cages among colonies of rats. As long as we kept them together in families in their spacious cages, nothing happened. When the males and females were segregated into equally spacious but separate cages, in each case a number of animals became infected. Strange clue! Could the social conditions of animals be one of the factors in the maintenance of their health? Was this 'straw' one indication of the direction in which we must look for health?[¶]

During the First World War he was in charge of a Field Ambulance Unit, was mentioned in Despatches and awarded the Military Cross.

From 1920 to 1926, he was Pathologist and Director of Pathological Studies at the Royal Free Hospital in London. Then until 1935 he was pathologist at the Ear, Nose and Throat Hospital and continued his research on the thyroid gland at Saint Bartholomew's Hospital with a grant from the Royal College of Surgeons, of which he was a member.

Scott Williamson's professional work involved the study of the biological laws that govern the progress in the body of diseases and disorders, but he continually pondered on the nature of the biological laws that govern *order* in the body – the order and harmony that is characteristic of health. He reflected on the body's power to maintain its wholeness, to repair damage to itself, to distinguish between friend and foe and to grow to the pattern contained in the seed at conception. He meditated on the relationship that exists throughout nature between a living being and its environment, and on that which exists between a living being and its

* *The Quality of Life* (Appendix no. 1)
† *ibid.*
¶ *ibid.*

component parts – its tissues, organs and cells. It appeared to him that in both cases the relationship is one of mutual sustenance: the part and the whole each acting in a way that is beneficial to the other.

Humans are a social species, and when Dr Williamson spoke of a person's environment he meant the social as well as the physical environment. He included the people with whom one is in contact. I shall do the same.

A man or a woman or a child is undeniably a living organism – a whole. But, Scott Williamson asked himself, what – apart from the total Earth's biosphere – are the greater wholes with which each human organism can be in a mutually health-promoting relationship? Could one of them be the family – in the first place, a woman and a man, later the couple and their children? Could another be the local community – the village or tribe or the neighbourhood of which the family is a part?

He pondered the question: Is the family a social whole that is potentially the greatest source of health in both the individual and society? Is woman plus man the essential human unit because, from such a unity, newness may be born, not only the child who is inevitably unique, but creativity of all kinds? Can this relationship of a man and a woman develop in both of them a more balanced and sane, less biassed or one-eyed outlook and, therefore, a truer awareness of reality? And can such a unit be a focus in human societies from which sanity and wisdom may radiate?

Scott Williamson was far from unobservant. He looked around him and saw that this idea of the family seemed to be more than a little unreal. Sometimes a family seemed to be merely a collection of individuals sharing the same roof and, occasionally, a meal; sometimes one individual dominated the rest of the family, overshadowing and stunting the growth of the rest; sometimes a family existed in a hot-house atmosphere into which the fresh air of the real world rarely penetrated; and frequently families had little contact with other families, so that parents and children had separate acquaintance, the parents only among their workmates and the children among their schoolmates, both meeting only people of their own generation. But he kept his faith in the potentiality of the family. He held on to his understanding of the nature of health and was constantly on the lookout for correspondences to it in internal and external family relationships. If he did not find them, he did not facilely conclude, 'This then is human nature.' Instead he reserved judgement, suspecting that it might be the largely man-made environment that is at fault, or that habits acquired through past conditioning, or the unsuspected presence of physical defects or deficiencies, or an unsuitable diet, might be responsible. Moreover, he wondered if the potentiality of the family for the nurturing of individuality and maturity fails to be realised if it can play no part in creating a greater whole, a larger human unit from which to draw sustenance in its turn. Does a family, particularly the small modern so-called 'nuclear' family, need to be in a mutually creative relationship with a neighbourhood community within which it can find – and unconsciously give – emotional, functional and intellectual nourishment?

If the answer to this question were to be 'Yes', all the more reason for trying to collect young families together. Another reason is more obvious: a person has a greater chance of achieving his potentiality for health if his environment is healthy from the very beginning of his life, so one must begin not with the child but with the family into which the child will be born; and try to create circumstances in which prospective parents can improve their health (in the comprehensive sense in which it is used in this book), and can have a chance to create a health-promoting environment for their children.

The group of young enthusiasts and the two doctors decided to begin by offering a health service in the form of a family club to all the families living in a selected area of London who were willing to pay a small membership subscription. Member-families would have the use of a club-room, a playroom for the children, a birth-control clinic, ante-natal, post-natal and infant welfare clinic, an orthopaedic clinic and an annual medical and dental inspection of every member of the family.

A search was made for an area of London housing families who were handicapped neither by extreme poverty nor by being supported on a pedestal of servants and bound by upper class social conventions. Within these limits, they wanted as much variety of income levels and occupations as possible. No part of central London seemed suitable, and the two doctors approached the Medical Officer of Health of the London Borough of Camberwell and told him of their plans. He said, 'There is little provision for infant welfare in the Borough. If you will be doing that, I shall be only too pleased to have you. Whatever else you do is nothing to do with me.' They told him that their aim was not to dispense charity, not to seek out the most helpless and unfortunate in order to succour them; that they were scientists hoping to find out how people living under modern industrial conditions of life might best cultivate health, and thus to benefit humankind as a whole. They asked him if he could recommend a fairly densely populated area of the Borough in which there were few unemployed or casual labourers, so that families would be reasonably well-nourished. He told them of a part of Peckham housing mainly steadily employed 'artisans' (skilled and semi-skilled workers and self-employed craftsmen), clerical workers, small business-men and tradesmen.

In April 1926, they took a small double-fronted house with a garden in Queen's Road, Peckham, which they furnished with a kitchen, club-room, consulting and changing rooms, childrens' playroom and, later, a bathroom. They circularised all households within easy walking – pram-pushing – distance of the club, inviting families – that is to say mated couples with or without children – to join the club, which they called The Pioneer Health Centre, having been forestalled by a food store in their first choice of name – The Health Centre. It was explained that it was not a treatment centre but was concerned with the promotion of health, and to detect the beginnings of disease and give advice as to how to procure any necessary treatment. There were only two conditions of membership: the payment of a family subscription of six old pence a week and periodic medical examination (or, as it was later called, 'health overhaul') for every member of the family.

Later, a large hut was built in the garden and was used for a playroom by the older children and for whist drives and dances. The club was open daily, except Sunday, from 2pm to 10pm. The doctors worked similar hours. Members were able to make appointments for the health overhaul to suit their convenience. The medical inspection was thorough: every part of the body was examined; specimens of blood, urine etc were collected for laboratory inspection. 'Nothing that we knew how to investigate clinically was omitted, for neither the individual nor the doctor was working under the pressure of the emergency of acute illness.'*

Scott Williamson and Innes Pearse were looking for health. They had chosen an area in which they expected to find relatively healthy people. They had stressed the fact that the club was not a place to come to for treatment and most of the people seeking membership maintained that they were well enough, 'in their usual health'. But what the two doctors *found* was sickness. They wrote, 'Of parents over twenty five years of age examined by us, we were greatly astonished to find that for all without exception there was something to be done and that in many there was frank disease.'†

Almost all the families were keen to obtain treatment for the disorders or diseases revealed; the two doctors and the social secretary were kept busy finding places where suitable treatment or diagnosis could be obtained.

Some knew they were ill but had not sought treatment for reasons, some of which would not apply at the present day with the easier access to a doctor or place of treatment that the NHS provides. But a larger number were quite unaware that anything was wrong. They were suffering from hidden disorders; and some of these were just as serious as the more manifest disorders. High blood pressure, tuberculosis, diabetes, cancer, are examples of disorders that can remain hidden for long periods. Pearse and Williamson wrote:

> All disease goes through the stage of being hidden in this way. The hidden stage may be rapid or may be long drawn out... The explanation

* 1931, p. 11
† *ibid.*

is to be found in principles of physiology. The body works on the basis of very large reserves held in store to cope with the demands made upon it by action and in emergency. If for any reason one organ begins to fail, other organs of the body, calling upon their special reserves, do 'overtime' as it were, to maintain an efficiency in the body as a whole. Technically they are said to 'compensate' for the initial deficiency. Indeed so efficiently is this done, more particularly in cases of insidious disease where slow transference of the load from one organ to the other is possible, that for long periods the presence of the disease may be entirely masked. All the patient can be aware of is a general inability to exert the same effort in emergency as formerly.*

They give an example:

A man of 39 had worked all his life on the tramways. He was a paviour. Laying stone sets between the tramlines on crowded thoroughfares for seventeen years or more, he had worked carefree and fearless of the traffic. Just about the time he and his wife joined the Pioneer Health Centre, he had become nervous of the traffic, and his wife it was who asked anxiously if the doctor thought anything could be done for her husband as she understood that if a man became nervous he was very prone to accident. At the medical overhaul, the husband himself complained of nothing except a slight morning cough; he considered 'nervousness' too trivial to speak to the doctor about. It was found that he had advanced emphysema (a condition of inelasticity of the lungs which diminishes their capacity for filling with air). Examination disclosed that this had overstrained the heart, although the breakdown point of neither lungs, heart nor the man's physical constitution generally had yet been reached. He was unaware of his physical disability; he only knew that he had lost the confidence he once had in himself. His former confidence was born of intuitive knowledge of reserves formerly entirely at his disposal in emergency. Disease had stealthily robbed him of these reserves. He was not aware of the disease but felt he could no longer cope with situations that might occur. Knowing of no reason for this state, he was nervous without reason, and therefore ashamed of being nervous. Only a trained observer could detect the disease and link the lack of confidence with the slow encroachment upon the man's functional reserves.†

A person may even be unaware of his lessening power of activity, for 'capacity for action seems frequently to determine the extent of the desire to act.' Some people suffering from hidden disorders tend to scale their lives down and draw in their horns without realising it. This means that they are not even tempted to do more than they can do without effort. As a result, their lives – and sometimes their families' lives too – become unnecessarily dull and stultifying.

They found that many people were suffering from 'established diseases', either manifest or hidden, and that almost all adults had one or

---

* 1931, p. 18
† *ibid.*, p. 19

more relatively minor ailments. People tended to adopt a fatalistic attitude to such things as corns, backache or indigestion, but these too could lead to a debilitating life-style and have unfortunate repercussions on the rest of the family.

> When these conditions are continuously present in parents, they tend to overshadow the home and thereby to limit the range of the child's environment...*

The relationship of the Doctors with the members of the Centre was, in many ways, like that of the country doctor of 100 years ago with the people living in the area of his practice. As he rode, or drove in his pony and trap on his rounds, he would stop and chat with the people he met, and he was able to observe them at work and play. Because of the friendly and leisurely manner in which the Centre doctors conducted the health overhaul, and because they were able to meet and observe them in the club-room and during the social occasions that the members organised for themselves, they came to know the families and the circumstances of their lives very well. This enabled them to be particularly helpful to parents who sought advice on infant and child welfare.

Many examples came to light of the far-reaching effects of trivial disorders, including psychological ones. They give an example of a simple misapprehension on the part of a man who, five years previously, had had an attack of influenza:

> During the attack, he had been told by his doctor that his heart was affected and that he must take care not to exert himself. This advice he followed. He became afraid to go out alone, afraid to go on a journey, afraid almost to laugh. On joining the Centre, he presented the appearance of a morose and sick man with one foot in the grave. His business had gone to pieces and he was casting the shadow of his supposedly imminent decease upon his adolescent family.
>
> On examination there were found to be no signs of heart disease present. Doubtless the heart, dilated during the influenzal attack when he was attending the doctor, had returned to normal size subsequently. The physical lesion had gone; the mental lesion had persisted. On being informed of the absence of any heart lesion and recommended to live an ordinary life, the man gathered courage, helped by his wife who took up the new cue with good sense and enthusiasm. They both entered into the life at the Centre, and, within two months, the man was once more leading an ordinary life. Not the least evidence of this was the fact that his business slowly began to flourish again.†

They found many cases of neuroses and depression with physical consequences in mothers struggling to rear children in totally unsuitable conditions and isolated with them throughout most of the 24 hours.

In the 1920s, community life still existed in parts of London. In the Borough of Poplar in London's dockland for instance, there was a social

* *ibid.*, p. 32
† *ibid.*, p. 152

life reminiscent of the English village before the industrial revolution, without the feudal superstructure.* The anonymity of city life had not yet taken over. In dockland, sons usually followed their father's trade; families lived for several generations in the same area and everyone was on at least nodding acquaintance with everyone else living in the same street. Photographs taken at this time in Poplar and in many country villages and small towns show that the street was still a centre of community life. They show adults conversing on their doorsteps while toddlers played at their feet. Older children played in the street with balls, tops and hoops or hopscotch and other traditional games; if they heard a vehicle approaching, they had plenty of time to skip out of the way and returned to their game after it had passed. (I remember in the village in which I grew up, the main road between the county town and another large town widened out as it passed through the centre of the village and the traffic went round the playing children; there was plenty of room for both.) In Poplar there was no nonsense about women being excluded from pubs: people remember the peas for the Sunday dinner being brought into the bar parlour to be shelled. In the summer, communally organised celebrations, fairs and festivities took place in the street. In such places in general, there was no need for anyone to be lonely, and help and sympathy were forthcoming in times of misfortune. No doubt one's business was not one's own only, but, at most stages of life, that is a small price to pay for a feeling of belonging to a community and for a familiar centre to one's life.

For the small child, in such a community, the world beckoned from beyond the kitchen door and he was often able to venture into it and to scuttle back to the shelter of mother or of some other well-known adult as he felt the need. Little children could be allowed out to play in the company of older ones when road traffic was slower and mostly confined to the most important thoroughfares. Sometimes the cobbler or the tailor working in his window would be aware of what was going on in the street or on the village green, and would intervene if serious danger threatened a child through his own or his playmates' ignorance. To a child growing up in such circumstances 'home' must have meant far more than the space between four walls where his parents ate and slept; it must have meant an increasingly rich and elaborate tapestry of characters and their occupations, of different family traditions and peculiarities, of the solidarity of the children as a group, of the warm refuge provided on occasion by a grandmother, an uncle, a neighbouring adolescent or older sister, besides a physical territory every inch of which was familiar to all his senses in its morning and evening and seasonal moods, because he had been free to explore it alone and at his leisure.

But Poplar was a backwater. Peckham, in contrast, was in the main twentieth century stream. The area around the Pioneer Health Centre was

* See Richman, 1975

much more like the inner city suburb of today, with a shifting population and no community feeling. Young people had left the districts in which they had grown up in order to find a job, or somewhere to set up house. Often husbands and wives had both moved right away from their families and friends. The women had also often left their jobs immediately on marriage, for married women were excluded from many jobs and professions. There seemed to be little opportunity for making friends. Usually one's workmates did not live locally and were therefore unknown to one's family. The same applied to schoolmates for those children who had won scholarships to a grammar school which might be at some distance. Although the many families living in two or three rooms in someone else's house did not think of themselves as particularly unfortunate or deprived, they did not choose to invite their neighbours into their home. There was loneliness and frustration particularly for young wives. So the opportunity the Centre offered to meet other women of an afternoon and chat for an hour or two while the children played in an adjoining room was eagerly seized on.

During the three years 1926 to 1929, 115 families (about 400 individuals) joined, and presented themselves for the health overhaul. Not all remained for the whole three years, but most were glad of the opportunity to exercise responsibility for their health and that of their families. The pilot scheme had answered in the affirmative the question: Are there families who would welcome information concerning the state of their physical fitness and who would take advantage of opportunities to improve it?

At first it was mostly young families with small children, or newly married couples, who joined the Centre. But, from about fifteen months after opening, older children and adolescents, attracted by something new and lively going on in the neighbourhood, began to bring their parents to the point of joining. From then on, the club premises began to feel cramped; it was increasingly difficult to provide for the social needs of people of such varied ages and tastes.

By 1929 it was plain that the premises were quite inadequate for a family health club. Although many of the schoolchildren and adolescents were suffering from 'nutritional deficiencies, structural defects and functional maladjustments', there were some who were mentally alert, physically energetic and full of enthusiasm and initiative.* There were members of all ages who, when their diseases or hidden disorders had been remedied, found themselves suddenly feeling the desire for a fuller life. Membership of the club did not give these people sufficient opportunity to satisfy their need for physical, mental and social activity. Also, it had become noticeable that many members, whose maladies had been successfully treated, relapsed and quickly developed the same or other troubles, and there were some people who, while not suffering from a

* 1931, p. 113

specific disease or disorder, had a lack of vitality which did not seem attributable to their physical condition and which seemed more likely to be accounted for by an environment that offered little opportunity for the exercise of their physical, mental and social faculties and the development of their potential talents. It was evident that the provision of medical examination and friendly consultation for the self-styled fit, although so necessary in the fight against disease, could not, by itself, promote health. Something was wrong with the circumstances of these peoples' lives and it was not, in many cases, shortage of cash. To change the environment of their working lives or their housing was too big an undertaking for a small group and too long-term, but to change their leisure-time environment was a possibility. It was evident that the club needed far larger premises, premises that were designed and equipped to allow people of all ages, from babies to the elderly, scope for their initiative, enterprise and social, physical and mental abilities – scope to grow. Health, Scott Williamson and Pearse had learned, implies growth. To stop growing is to begin to die.

For three years the Doctors had been learning the extent of the ill-health of the inhabitants of Peckham, and had been engaged in finding solutions to their individual problems; but they had also been learning more about the basic biological needs of human beings. Although sickness and lack of vitality constantly forced themselves on their attention, they were always on the look-out for manifestations of health, and, because they obtained an increasingly clearer idea of what they were looking for, they were able to recognise it when they saw it. They saw manifestations of health in the high spirits of some of the children, although, for lack of suitable situations in which to exercise it, it often resulted in anti-social behaviour. They saw it sometimes in young couples in love, seeing the world anew through each others' eyes, and full of new vitality; although this was often an ephemeral phenomenon, not only because of the social poverty in which they lived but also because of the attitude of the pair to marriage, the young man tending to wear his wife like an emblem on his sleeve or a flower in his buttonhole, and the young woman feeling that, with marriage, she had obtained her object in life and had reached the stage in the story when they would 'live happily ever after'. They saw it in the babies and toddlers, single-minded in their devotion to the satisfaction of their urge to develop their human powers – walking, talking and innumerable other mental, physical and social skills. They saw it in the pleasure of the club members of all ages in meeting familiar faces in the club-room and in their responsive and responsible attitude to each other. They saw it in the strong desire of most parents to do their utmost for their children's happiness and welfare, often at considerable self-sacrifice; although what was done was sometimes not at all in the best interests of the child. In Peckham at that period, there was a tendency towards small families: people were determined not to subject their children to the privations they themselves had suffered through having too many siblings. Many found themselves spending all the money they could spare on presents for their one or two children and giving them so much of their time and attention that their own mental growth suffered. As a result they had less and less to offer the child in the way of nourishment for his powers of thought and feeling. If parents turn their backs on the world and focus all their attention on the child, he or she will tend to become self-absorbed and egoistic simply for lack of anything other than himself with which to be concerned.

The decision was taken to close the first Pioneer Health Centre and to design and collect funds for a new and purpose-built Centre.

In a new Centre, it was hoped that parents, children, young people and the elderly would be able to share their leisure without treading on each others' toes. It was hoped to alleviate to some extent the effect of twentieth century conditions of life where people are segregated according to age, where the parents' working – and, sometimes, leisure – lives are far from the ken and understanding of the children, and where children spend the day being 'minded' with others of precisely similar age in a world of school they find impossible to describe to parents, so that the family does not act as an aid to digestion of the child's experience, and the child is unable to involve other members of the family in his interests, projects and friendships. And it was hoped that, in a new Centre, the conditions in which health could flower, and in which the biological laws that govern health would freely operate, could be recognised and defined.

The two doctors and their supporters set about publicising their project. In 1931, the Pioneer Health Centre became registered with the Board of Charity Commissioners for England and Wales as 'a company not having a share capital and limited by guarantee'. The executive committee of the company set out to find financial support for the project. The money was slow to come in, because the current economic slump was at its height; this caused the committee of the PHC some anxiety. Then Jack Donaldson (later Lord Donaldson of Kingsbridge) joined the group and, soon afterwards, transferred £10,000 of the £22,000 he had inherited from his father to the account of the Pioneer Health Centre. This generous action inspired others to give on a larger scale than before, and another £10,000 was immediately subscribed. They had then enough money for the building that Scott Williamson had designed, and, when a site in St Mary's Road, a turning off Queen's Road, Peckham, was made available to them, they decided to go ahead and errect it, while continuing to seek funds to cover the running costs of the club while the membership was building up. Lord Nuffield contributed generously at this time.

It was calculated that the Centre would be self-supporting with a membership of 2,000 families. The weekly family subscription would be one shilling. Adults would be charged a few pence for the use of amenities such as the swimming pool, billiards tables and badminton court. Tea, coffee, beer, cider and light refreshments would be sold in the self-service cafeteria. Only money for research would still be sought from outside; for example, members would not be expected to pay for experimental trials of dietary supplements such as iron and vitamins.

The new Pioneer Health Centre was opened in May, 1935.

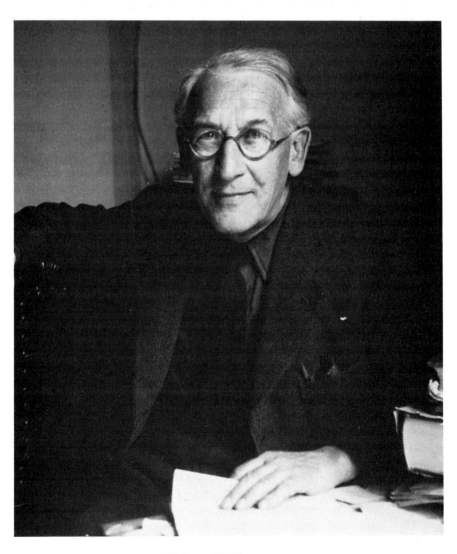

G Scott Williamson

Chapter 2

Four Essential Conditions of the Experiment

Half a century ago, Scott Williamson used the word 'ethology' to describe the area of knowledge in which he worked. His definition was 'the study of the state of order and ease which is the opposite of the state of disorder and disease that is called "pathology"'. Today, 'ethology' is used to mean the study of the behaviour of animals in their natural environment.

The natural environment of animals is one in which they have proved to be successful and have long survived and flourished because it answers their needs. Therefore, if an ethologist is to learn anything about the true nature of the human animal, he must be able to observe its behaviour in an environment that answers its basic needs. The new Centre was to be an attempt to provide – within a modern industrial society – environmental conditions that would answer the needs of human beings as a species. 'Needs', Scott Williamson might have defined as the possibility of realising one's physical, mental and social potential to the full.

Students of human ethology is a true description of Doctors Pearse and Williamson; but, even today, ethology is not a commonly used word and I shall give them the title they gave themselves – 'biologists'. This, in fact suits them better, because it not only describes them as workers but as thinkers: they were aware of the world as a living whole and of people as living wholes, with all that that implies.

The main conditions created by the 'Peckham Biologists' that made it possible for the inhabitants of an area of Peckham in the second quarter of the twentieth century to satisfy their needs in this sense were, in my opinion, five in number:

1. The building
2. The health overhauls and consultations
3. The family and local membership
4. The financial contribution of the families to the Centre
5. The careful maintenance of a 'strict anarchy'.

This chapter contains a description of the first four of these.

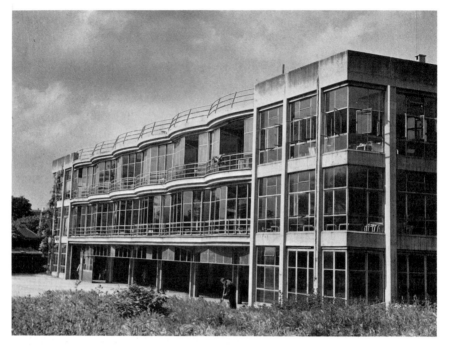

The Peckham Health Centre

The building

This was designed by Scott Williamson together with Owen Williams (later Sir E Owen Williams). It was described by one of the leading architects of the time, Walter Gropius, as 'an oasis of glass in a desert of brick'. It is a building that still satisfies the eye, and has been officially 'listed' as a building to be preserved.

Advantage was taken of the building techniques and materials that make it possible to do without weight-bearing walls and thus to make it easy for people to see and to move from one part of the building into another. The design was open-plan, but it did not dwarf the human being; it encouraged one to loiter and, even when on one's own, to feel neither lonely nor self-conscious.

In architectural terms, it consisted of three large concrete platforms, (160 x 120 feet) one above the other, cantilevered widely over supporting pillars arranged in parallel series, surrounding a rectangular central space occupied by a swimming pool (35 x 75 feet). The deep end of the pool rested on the ground and the water was level with the first floor. There was a continuous glass 'window' along both sides of the pool so that one could see into it from almost any part of the first floor and right through it from the back to the front of the building and to the trees outside. The glass roof of the pool chamber was high and steeply pitched in order to carry off the noise. An apparatus was installed that removed water vapour and helped prevent condensation on the glass surround.

The design of the building was strictly functional, inside and out. No money was wasted on decoration, yet it was an aesthetically pleasing, elegant building. The entrance was far from grandiose. One walked past the gatekeeper's hut, along the wire netting that fenced in the playground, to the back of the building. Inside on the right, a concrete staircase led up to the main social floor; on the left was a pram and bicycle park and the door to the boiler room and the haunts of the maintenance engineer; ahead a broad passage with the entrance to the theatre/badminton court on the right and on the left the way in to the swimming pool and the gymnasium via the toilets and changing rooms. There were also four 'slipper baths' (much appreciated in the 1930s) on this side of the passage which ended in a door leading to the partly covered children's playground, at the end of which was the glass fronted, downstairs children's nursery.

Arriving on the first floor, one was greeted by light, space and movement, even when, early in the afternoon, the building might be almost empty. The southern wall was entirely of glass, but the daylight glare was broken by the gently angled window bays and again by the widely spaced pillars of smooth grey concrete that supported the upper floors. The effect of movement was caused by the light shining down from the roof and reflecting from the rippling water of the pool.

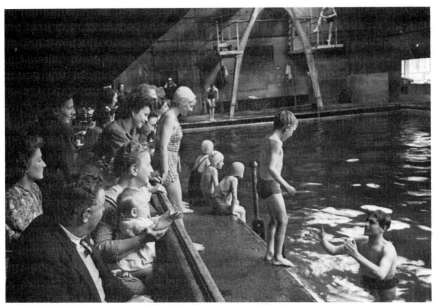

For a brief period after the War, there was no glass between the cafeteria and the swimming pool

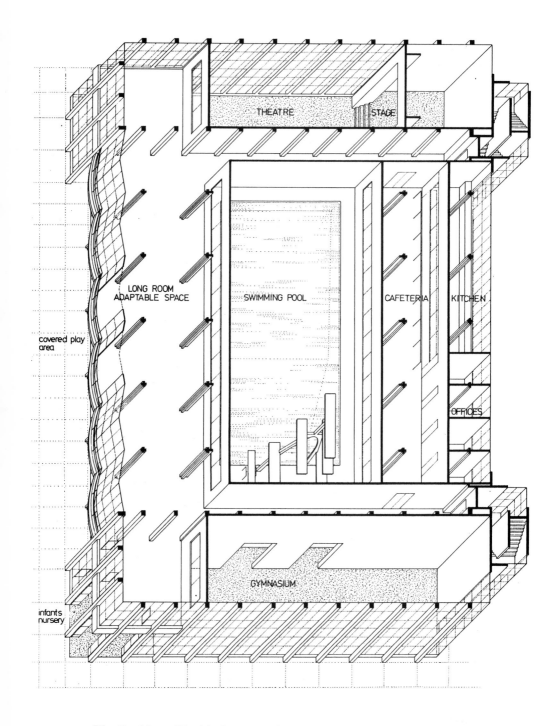

The Peckham Health Centre – first floor and parts of ground floor

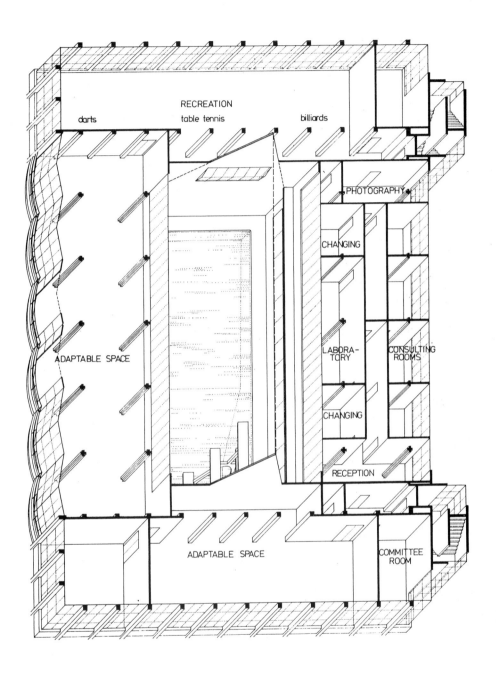

The Peckham Health Centre – second floor

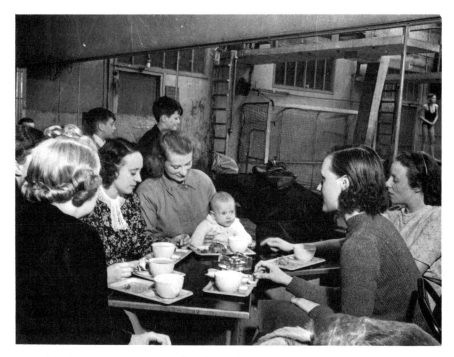

In the cafeteria

One could sit and watch the swimmers and divers from the chairs and tables that lined the glass surround of the pool both on the northern (cafeteria) side and in the long gallery-like hall known as the Long Room that ran the whole length of the building on the south side. The tables and chairs were designed brilliantly by a young architect, Christopher Nicholson, who was shortly afterwards tragically killed in a gliding accident in mist over the Alps. Their design reflected the shape of the cruciform pillars between which they were placed, solid but not at all heavy in aspect. The tables were designed to seat the maximum number of people in a small space. The chair was made of a single sheet of thick plywood and padded with foam rubber, and was comfortable, good to look at and, like the tables, economical of space. At either end of the Long Room on its inner side were fifteen feet wide glass 'viewing windows' through which one could see down into the gymnasium and the theatre/badminton court which occupied spaces two storeys high.

From the street at night, the building shone with a welcoming light. The Long Room was particularly suitable for festive social gatherings but also for cosy meetings between acquaintances, because the spaces between the pillars supporting the upper storey formed alcoves along both the window and the pool sides that invited relaxed conversation. As one-time members recall, these alcoves served many useful purposes – a small birthday celebration for instance, or a place in which the shy or those who wanted to watch what was going on in the pool or on the dance floor without too obviously doing so or drawing attention to themselves could shelter. Young teenagers often availed themselves of this opportunity. The polished cork tiles covering the floors were ideal for dancing. The unadorned concrete and cork afforded a restful and neutral background in a building usually full of people, and, to my mind, it was attractive even when empty. In order to deaden noise in a building intended to accommodate 1,000 or more active individuals of all ages at one time, cork was also used to cover walls and ceilings, the last covered with a colour wash.

The authors of *The Peckham Experiment* note in an appendix that:

... four years' experience has shown the completely satisfactory nature of the ceiling and floor surfaces. Cork as a wall covering reduces the noise factor, but while admirably suited to the 'medical' department, has proved unsatisfactory in other parts of the building owing to the attractive surface it offers to the penknives of the idle newcomer... Particular mention should be made of the construction of the special floors designed by Scott Williamson for the gymnasium and the theatre (used also for Badminton and for dancing). Across an unscreeded concrete base, $1/2$" rubber $1/8$" bore pressure tubing was stretched in parallel lines. The space intervening between the lines of tubing (9 to 12 inches according to the degree of spring required) was then filled in with cork chips till level with the summit of the tubing. The level surface thus formed was covered with the same tongued and grooved cork squares as the other

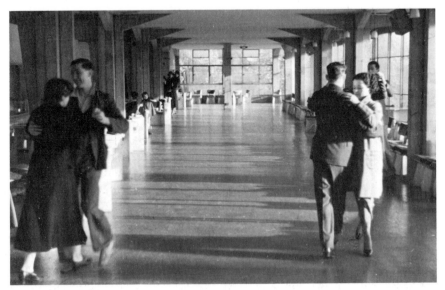

The Long Room

floors in the building. The effect of this construction was to give a uniform resilience, with a softness and a gentle spring not unlike turf, and without dead areas due to joists. This floor surface proved over $4^1/_2$ years' continuous use to have an excellent wearing capacity.'

The building has been well-cared for by its present users, the Inner London Education Authority; but they have replaced the cork with other wall and ceiling covering and conversation is now difficult when the place is crowded. They have also divided it up into rooms and destroyed the easy access to every part of the building.

Throughout, there was a pleasant absence of blank-walled corridors and closed doors. The only enclosed part of the building, apart from a committee room or two used also for listening to music or Dance Band practice, was the Consultation Block, popularly referred to as the 'medical department', which took up less than a quarter of the top floor. It included a small reception and waiting room, consulting rooms, changing cubicles and a laboratory.

Close to the Consultation Block, in a lightly partitioned off part of the long sunny hall that was a replica of the 'Long Room' on the floor below, was the babies' and toddlers' nursery; and, in a corner of it, with a window overlooking the nursery, was the doctor's consultation room for mothers and babies.

The more effectively mobile of the under-fives were promoted to the nursery on the ground floor, adjacent to the outdoor playground and to

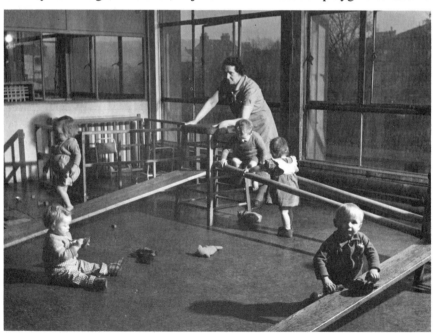

the gymnasium and small 'learners' pool. This last was situated between the concrete tank of the main swimming pool and the gymnasium. It was about 8 feet wide and 25 feet long and was filled slowly each day, so that by 4.30 in the afternoon it was deep enough for an adult to learn in, while at 2.30, the depth of the water was a mere six to ten inches. Except during school holidays, a number of the older and more capable of the nursery children were allowed into the gym and the learners' pool, under close supervision, early in the afternoon, before the school-age children flocked in.

The space used for nurseries in the afternoons was available for adult use in the evenings. The exception was the ground floor nursery in which babies who could still sleep comfortably in their perambulators could be left, between 8pm and 10.30pm, in the charge of a nursery nurse.

The billiards tables (two full-size and a smaller one for the children's use), table-tennis tables and darts boards were on the top floor at the western end of the building.

The kitchen, with its self-service counter where tea, coffee, beer, cider, snacks and supper dishes could be bought by members, was on the northern side of the cafeteria. It was entirely visible from the service counter, from which people helped themselves – and queued if necessary, so the cooking and preparation of dishes went on in full view of the members. Next to it was the small office with its hatch at which one could pay one's weekly family membership subscription. Here also, for three old pence, members could obtain a metal disk for use in the turnstiles at the entrances to the men's and women's changing rooms for the pool and gymnasium, and, for two old pence, borrow a key to one of the slipper baths.

The cafeteria became the main gathering point in the building and, at times during the evening, it became very crowded. It was hard on the members of staff who were bound to be in or near the office, taking subscriptions or being available. This was almost the only defect in a building that proved to have been designed almost perfectly for its purpose.

For the purpose of facilitating spontaneous participation in activities of all kinds and the practice of self-service, the design could not have been bettered. The number of servicing and administrative staff found to be necessary was very small indeed. People wandered freely everywhere and were able to see what there was to do and who was doing it without, as in a community centre I know, having to peer through a small glass door panel. Even if their intention on entering the building had been merely to enjoy a coffee or a beer in a friendly social atmosphere, they found movement and activity all around them. It was easy also to locate one's friends or the members of one's family if they were in the building, and for companionship to be a matter of choice and not merely chance.

The design also enabled the Biologists to observe the use made of the Centre by member-families, with whom they had already become acquainted in the course of their duties in the consultation block or elsewhere in the building. Incidentally these duties left them no time – even if they had had the tactlessness to do so – to stand about, pencil and notebook in hand; but it was easy for them to notice what was going on when seizing a free moment to take a stroll around, or when taking their tea and supper breaks in the cafeteria.

I find it difficult to imagine a health-promoting club on the lines of the Peckham Centre operating successfully in a different kind of building. The design of the building was one of the factors that made possible the growth of the all-age community. It made it possible for children and adults to find their own chosen amusements within sight of each other, for the younger to find acceptance with the older and to learn from them consciously and unconsciously, and for young families to benefit from interaction with families at a later stage of development, and it helped all to discover their own tastes and abilities and to fulfil their potential for mature development.

The health overhauls and consultations

The health overhaul was in three parts. First a visit to the laboratory for biochemical tests, including blood and urine analysis. Sight and hearing were tested, height and weight measured, blood pressure taken, a spirometer reading made and arterial tone recorded on the Plesch tonoscillograph.

After this, an appointment with the doctor was made for two or three days later when the results of the laboratory tests would have become available. The doctors and laboratory staff worked from 2pm to 10pm including Saturdays but not Mondays. The Centre building was open every day except Sunday from 2pm until 10.30pm and 11pm on Saturday. Females and all children under seven were examined by a woman doctor. The medical staff consisted of two men and two women. The Consultation block was staffed also by a biochemist and his assistant, a trained nurse and a receptionist. For the examination by the doctor, each person was asked to strip, having been shown into a changing cubicle and handed a freshly sterilised long white gown and warm dressing gown to put on. Every part of the body was examined and posture and gait noted. The Centre doctors' aim was not to elicit symptoms or detect diseases, but to 'estimate the direction, the degree and the perfection of the function of the body in action'. Little was said on this occasion, as information and discussion were reserved for the family consultation which followed at a time when all the family could forgather to meet the two doctors who had examined the individual members of the family.

The doctor who had examined the youngest child would begin this consultation by giving the results of its laboratory tests and physical examination in ordinary non-medical language wherever possible, with the emphasis on what was right rather than on what was wrong. Each child in turn left the room after the results of his or her overhaul had been gone through, until the parents were left alone with the two doctors and could discuss any problems concerning the children's condition more fully. Then the results of the parents' overhauls were given and discussed. In the relaxed and leisurely atmosphere of the consultation, anxieties, fears and hopes were brought to the surface and expressed; experience, facts and knowledge were looked at by the couple and the doctors together. The family consultation was a

> ... means of giving to the family and all its individuals the facts that were gathered from the health overhaul and of passing such facts through the family mill for digestion.*

A few months after the opening of the St Mary's Road Centre, Mary Langman, the Biologist's private secretary, was typing in the laboratory when a Centre member came up with a family she was showing round, and asked her to say something about the family consultation. Miss Langman repeated what she had heard the doctors say, that no treatment was given – only advice. At this the member interrupted with, 'No, that's quite wrong; they don't give you advice; they tell you how you stand.' Evidently, there had been a change in the Biologists' methods. This was not surprising since the technique of the family consultation was still being worked out.

The appropriate technique must necessarily be different from that used by a medical practitioner who is consulted by a 'patient' hoping to be relieved of suffering and incapacity and, who is willing to put himself entirely into the doctor's hands. The relationship was not that of professional and patient; it was more that of a professional and a client, although that is also an incorrect description because the Centre members were initially not even seeking advice. The families had not joined the Centre because they were ill or wanted help with their lives; they did not come to the Centre doctors as patients, and many of them would not have taken kindly to being treated as such. (A member, Gladys Coring, told me, 'If they had said, "You do this and the other," I would have backed off at once.') But, as Williamson and Pearse say, 'To anyone trained in the medical profession – that is, specifically to give advice – it is extremely difficult not to do so... We try to refrain from assuming the authority of special knowledge.'

* 1943

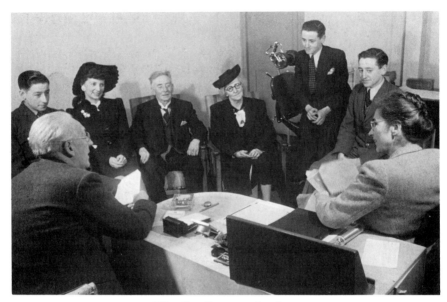

The family consultation

At the first family consultation, the Biologists attempted to lay the foundations of a friendly and easy relationship, based on mutual respect. This approach was essential for, in order to promote the health they sought to study, it was necessary to act in a manner that would strengthen a person's faith in himself – his faith in his own common sense and deepest feelings. The members valued the full and honest information given to them, the doctors' recognition of their right and ability to decide for themselves what – if anything – to do about it, their easy availability and approachability and their willingness to share, like a true friend, their knowledge and wisdom when needed.

The members did not get the feeling that they were being graded and pigeon-holed, because Scott Williamson and Innes Pearse did not label people 'healthy' or less than healthy in different degrees, even in their own minds. In the first place, they knew that health had to do with quality and was therefore difficult – perhaps impossible – to measure; secondly they knew that it could be manifested in as many different ways as there are people; thirdly they had found that people could be apparently free of physical disorders and deficiencies and yet lack vitality. Above all, they did not think of health as a state; they thought of it as a way of acting, a way of relating with the environment. To them the growth of capability, spontaneity, autonomy and responsibility were all manifestations of health. But these powers cannot grow in entirely unsuitable surroundings; the quality of a person's relationship with his environment at any moment must be to some extent dependent on the quality of his environment at that moment.

This means that a person's health can never be assessed independently of his social and physical environment.

On bidding goodbye to the family at the end of the family consultation, the doctors reminded them that they could, at any time, ask the receptionist for an appointment with one or other of the doctors if they wanted to discuss anything further or if they were worried by anything, even the apparently trivial.

A pregnancy was of primary interest to the Biologists; a 'parental consultation' was offered to any couple whose pregnancy was confirmed and when the woman had had her laboratory check-up to see if her physiological reserves were as high as possible. As with all family consultations, the man and woman Biologists were both present. The consultation began with a review of the wife's recent check-up. The results were explained and, if she and her husband were interested, any necessary remedial action was discussed. Innes Pearse describes the nature of the overhauls and various family consultations very fully in *The Peckham Experiment* and *The Quality of Life*.

During pregnancy, laboratory tests were available to the woman fortnightly and a consultation with the woman doctor and the nurse monthly.

The babies' nursery was next to the consultation block and the nurse in charge welcomed prospective mothers in for a chat. She would answer their questions and they could make the acquaintance of the babies. Thus, by the time a woman found herself responsible for the care of her own, she would feel a little more confident in her ability. Babies would no longer be quite strange and alien creatures.

The Peckham Biologists considered pregnancy and the birth of the baby to be matters that concerned both parents equally, and that, when they both felt involved, these experiences could mature them both. They held that pregnancy, like puberty and mating, is one of the important 'biological junctions', when a person can change direction as it were. 'The pregnancy is important, not only because of the coming of the baby, but because of all it can do for you yourselves.' They would add that at this time it is important that the circumstances of one's life should be favourable for development – for the widening of interests, the making of friends and the development of talents. 'Pregnancy is no one-way process in which, as it used to be thought, you had to sacrifice yourself for the baby's sake. On the contrary, it is a mutual process between you and your baby, a process by which each benefits the other.'*

In *The Peckham Experiment* (p. 153) there is a lyrical description of how, when a woman's diet is suitable, her life active and her attitude one of confidence, her body builds up reserves of energy and material that become available as needed during pregnancy so that she feels full of energy and, at the end, she is 'like an athlete in training awaiting the starting pistol, attuned to maximum effort yet relaxed'.

* 1979, p. 53

It was explained to the family why the expectant mother's diet was especially important and they were told about the fresh vegetables and fruit and the 'live' TT milk from the Centre's farm that were on sale in the cafeteria and reserved, in the first place, for families with – or expecting – babies.

Then, or at a later consultation, the couple's curiosity about the birth process was satisfied. After the war, as Dr Pearse described, she 'was fortunate in having a copy of the admirable *Birth Atlas* produced for the Maternity Centre of New York'. With its help, she said, it was easy to run through the stages of pregnancy from the beginning to the wonderful way in which the healthy body makes provision for the birth. The couple might be told, for example, of the recent discovery that a few hours before the onset of labour, there occur changes in the fluid-content of a woman's tissues and the loosening up of her joints and cartilages that render them more malleable and expansile. Often the pair were filled with wonder and began to look forward with pleasure to the birth itself and not only to the moment when it would be over.

The place of birth was discussed. At a time when, in this country, it was considered advisable for the birth of a baby to be followed by the 'confinement' of the mother to her bed for a fortnight or so, Innes Pearse blazed a new trail. Many of the mothers of babies conceived during membership of the Centre were so full of vitality and energy during pregnancy that it was patently absurd suddenly at the time of delivery to treat them as sick people requiring hospitalisation or confinement to bed. The Peckham Biologists felt that for a mother to be forced to deliver her baby in a place in which she is regarded and treated as a 'patient' was not only absurd; it was detrimental to health. At this peak moment in her life, she should be completely mistress of herself and of her surroundings and she should be able to share the event with whom she chooses. At this time, as mothers know well, a woman is particularly sensitive to events and to her surroundings, and her experiences during and immediately after the birth may affect her deeply and colour the rest of her life. Dr Pearse made an arrangement with the neighbouring King's College Hospital for a 48-hour admission for Centre members who had remained free from disorder and deficiencies during their pregnancy. This was the first arrangement of its kind in the country. To Dr Pearse this was not the ideal, but most of the younger families lived in unsuitable conditions for a 'home birth' (no running water in the apartment for example). For this reason or because the wife was not disorder-free or because she preferred to go into hospital, Dr Pearse was very rarely able to recommend delivery at home.

Parents welcomed the 48-hour arrangement for it allowed them to enjoy their baby's early days in the peace and privacy of their own homes and to be visited by the Centre nurse whom they already knew well; but, as Mrs Purser has recalled,* some of them did not enjoy the two days they spent in hospital.

It was often noticed that couples who had made good use of the Centre during the pregnancy would come in only rarely for a few weeks after the birth, preferring to stay at home with their baby although they could have brought it to the Centre and left it in the charge of the nursery nurse either during the afternoon or the evening. It seemed to the Biologists as if, at this time, parents have an instinct to retire from the public gaze and outside responsibilities and to be alone with the baby. The Peckham Biologists held that this 'centripetal phase' of family action is, like the similar honeymoon period, an important formative period for the family organism. Confinements in hospital can, they felt, deprive families of a great opportunity for the deepening of family relationships and for the maturing of both the woman and the man that this crucial moment in their lives can bring. Dr Pearse once remarked that a bonus that comes with a home birth is that a previously youngest or 'only' child can feel implicated in the arrival of the new baby, and, by the time friends and neighbours call, can proudly introduce them to 'our baby'.

Usually one or both parents brought the new baby for its first visit to the laboratory at a few days old. After this, another parental consultation was offered, and yet another at the weaning stage.

Mothers were invited to bring the baby weekly at first and then fortnightly to the afternoon baby clinic. These services included routine laboratory tests. It was much appreciated, not least because one could be sure of always seeing the same doctor (or occasionally the other of the two women doctors on the staff).

If the parents wished, they could bring toddlers to the woman doctor monthly, children from three to five at three-monthly intervals and school children could have an overhaul every six months.

The wellbeing of a small child can be more fully appraised by observing its behaviour and noting the quality of its play. At the Centre, the babies' and toddlers' spontaneously chosen play in the nurseries could easily be observed by parents and the doctor together and the knowledge of children's growth and development obtained in this way was usually very welcome to the parents.

Whenever the mother wished and however young the baby, she could leave it in the nursery while she enjoyed some recreation elsewhere in the building for an hour or two. Later, as the child grew, many mothers used the nurseries for the child's sake as well as for their own. I shall tell more about the nurseries elsewhere in the book.

Some young couples asked for pre-conception overhauls, in order to ascertain that they were as fit as possible before beginning a baby. Before long there was a demand for pre-marital overhauls.

* See Chapter 8

Children under 16 automatically became members when their parents joined and were entitled to use, without payment, all the amenities that were open to children. Children over 16 living at home could join the Centre if they wished, paying a weekly subscription equal to half the family one. A steady boy or girl friend could be enrolled as a temporary member, for a similar subscription. Temporary members were entitled to use all the amenities of the Centre, paying, like all adults, a small sum on each occasion, but did not get an overhaul. If, however, the pair became engaged to marry, and had fixed the date of the wedding, they could ask for a pre-marital overhaul and were treated as a new family. The content of the pre-marital family consultations varied to some extent from family to family because the Biologists usually knew at least one of the pair very well.

The family and local membership

As the reader will later learn, members of the Centre appreciated more than anything the fact that the whole family could use the Centre, could have the benefit of the health overhaul and the family consultation, and could find – and make – occupations to their taste. One former member described it as 'a place that *all* the family enjoyed and never tired of'. Because of its popularity with the children, parents, unable themselves to spend the whole afternoon or evening there, had the satisfaction of knowing where their children were, and of knowing they were happily occupied and relatively safe. Although membership was strictly a family one, use of the Centre was individual. Most of the children of the member families came to the Centre on their own, either straight from school or, on holidays, from home, at any time after the Centre opened at 2pm. Some would meet their mothers at the Centre and, at the end of the afternoon, go home together, having collected the baby or the toddler from the nursery. Children of secondary school age usually came on their own later, having done their homework and had a bite to eat first. From about 6pm to 8pm, they had the building virtually to themselves. Within that period, the staff took their supper break as it was the least popular time for appointments with the Doctors.

Saturday afternoon was the commonest time for a family to come in all together, but if a father was a shiftworker he might also be in the building at the same time as the children on a weekday afternoon.

Sometimes a man had such long hours of work that he could not make much use of the Centre, and some were studying in the evenings or attending evening classes, but were glad that their families should benefit. Many couples made the most of Saturday evening – usually quite a festive occasion. Sometimes a husband and wife ran a family business which they could not leave together, or they had difficulty in

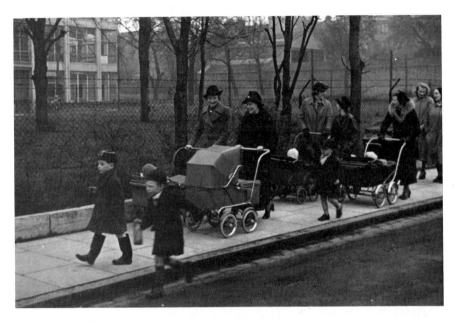

'all within walking distance'

finding baby sitters, and so they had to use the Centre separately, but the Centre was known to them both; it was common ground to the family; everyone, adult or child, could talk about what he or she had done there and be understood by the others. Husband and wife, parents and children could share their leisure-time experience, often as never before.

The family-membership rule made for continuity of membership and, therefore, continuity of acquaintanceships and a balance of the sexes and of age groups. Children and parents could not only share their leisure-time experiences but also their friends. The children made the acquaintance of their parents' friends and of their friends' families, and whole families formed lasting friendships. The situation was not unlike that in the extended family where there is likely always to be someone a little older or younger than oneself with whom to relate, instead of the gulf of twenty or thirty years between two generations. Without the family membership rule, the all-age community life which distinguished the Centre would have been most unlikely to have come about. The causes of this happy mingling of parents of all ages, teenagers, old people and children – or rather its apparent causes – are described in a later chapter, but the family membership was certainly one of the enabling circumstances.

How much of this was foreseen by the founders is impossible to say, but family membership had been a part of their plan from the very first: it was a necessary condition for the research they intended to do. In their

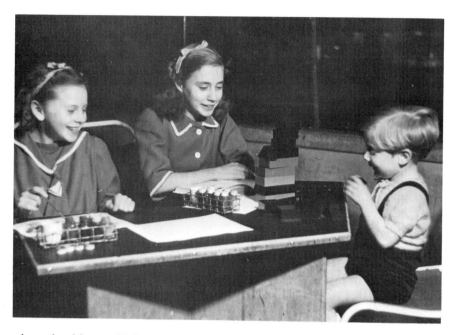

view, health could best be observed and studied in a community of families, where the unit is the mated pair with or without children.

Families were only eligible for membership if they lived within a designated area around St Mary's Road known as 'the District'. It was of a rather irregular shape due to the barriers formed by the railway lines (which cover London, south of the river, in curving patterns) and by a main road. The furthest corners of the District were within little more than a mile of the Centre. This was manageable by pram-pushing parents, and young children. The local residence rule made for regular and frequent use of the Centre by the members and for individual use by every member of the family. Motor traffic within the District in the thirties and forties was not heavy and most of the children could safely make their own way to the Centre.

If membership had been open to individuals and had had no residential qualifications, the Centre might have acquired a full membership very quickly, but people, especially those free of family responsibilities, would have been likely to join for the sake of one amenity only – the health overhaul or the swimming pool and gymnasium perhaps. It could have become filled by young sports enthusiasts or middle-aged hypochondriacs from far afield, with the result that the people living in the neighbourhood who wanted to make it the social centre of their lives would have been crowded out.

At the Centre, members and Biologists might meet casually and informally at any time, but one more formal meeting remains to be

described. This was the 'enrolment talk'. Often a family would be introduced to the Centre by an existing member-family, who would show
them round the building; otherwise, a member of staff would do so or
would ask a member – known to be willing – to do so. The tour always
ended with the Consultation block. There the family were introduced to
the receptionist, with whom they could make an appointment to meet the
Doctors for an enrolment talk, in which, they were told, they could hear
more about the Centre and its purpose, before deciding whether or not to
join.

At this interview, whenever her duties allowed, one other member of
the scientific staff was present – the Biologist on the social floor. During
the pre-war period, this post was held by Lucy H Crocker, co-author of
The Peckham Experiment. After the war, she was, for a year or two,
unfortunately unable to rejoin the staff as she was living far from
London with her husband and two small children. Her position was
described – entirely accurately – as the 'curator of the instruments of
health'. It was to her that members or groups of members came to book
space for activities they wished to initiate; she also supervised the activity of the children in the afternoons and early evenings and saw to it
that any equipment that they were authorised to use was available to
them. Lucy Crocker became a very valuable member of Williamson's
and Pearse's team. Indeed when I speak of the Peckham Biologists, it is
principally to these three that I am referring.

At the enrolment talk, the family were informed of conditions of
membership. These were two – firstly an undertaking to pay a weekly
subscription which covered all the overhauls and consultations, use of
the nurseries, and use of all the amenities of the club by children under
sixteen, and secondly an undertaking that every member of the family
would submit to an overhaul on joining and then annually. An excerpt
from the Annual Report of the Pioneer Health Centre for 1936 gives an
idea of the information that was given to prospective member-families:

> On looking round the Centre, you may have thought it was a place of
> amusement. It is that, but it is also much more, for its chief purpose is to
> maintain the health of the adults and to develop the health of their
> children. It is a Health Centre. It is not concerned with sickness and that
> is why we undertake no treatment. The Health Doctor, just like the
> Sickness Doctor, needs his tools but they are of a very different kind.
> They are those things you see as you go round the Centre: the gymna-
> sium, the swimming bath, the nursery, the cafeteria, the dance floor, and
> so on, and many more will be devised as the Centre grows. It is natural
> that the instruments for health should be varied because health covers a
> very wide field, and includes physical, mental, social and even economic
> life.
>
> If the service offered is to be of value to its members it must be
> conducted in an orderly and scientific way and not by guess-work. That

is why we ask all our members to come periodically for a health over-haul, so that the facts that have been discovered about each family may be put before them to use as they think best. All examinations are fixed at times to suit the convenience of the members, appointments being made any time between 2 and 10 p.m. daily. Sundays and Mondays excepted.

We then explain that the Centre was built by private people who wanted to find a means whereby the more recent advances in Science could be made available for the use of the average person. The service has been so planned that when there are enough member-families it will become self-supporting. The staff, including the doctors, will then be paid servants of the members, with no intervening loyalties to undermine mutual confidence. This point is always immediately appreciated, especially by the father.

It follows that the Centre, catering as it does for all wage levels, including the lowest, can only exist by cutting down expenditure to a minimum. And since service is the most expensive item, we must work toward the time when the scientific and technical staff will be the only paid servants. This implies the development of self-service throughout the building; but if the Centre is looked on as an extension of one's home – one's own billiard room, one's own nursery, the place where one entertains one's friends – this is easy to understand.

If the family decided immediately to join, they proceeded to pay their first weekly family subscription and to make their individual appointments for the laboratory tests.

The financial contribution of member-families to the running of the Centre

'Health and responsibility are synonymous,' wrote Pearse and Williamson.* Healthy action is action that is responsive to the needs both of oneself and of one's surroundings. It is responsible action. It follows that if one wishes to promote health in a society, one must try to create conditions in which responsibility for oneself and one's environment is possible. Scott Williamson held that being the recipient of charity curbs one's capacity for responsible actions – even if there are no obvious strings attached and the donor is the taxpayer. He felt very strongly that the member-families should pay for what they got, but, since he wanted to include people from all walks of life in his experiment, the rate at which they were asked to pay should be no higher than those with low incomes could manage. The weekly family subscription was fixed at one shilling, plus six old pence for every child over 16 living at home who wished to belong. In addition an adult paid three old pence for each swim or use of any other facility or three or six old pence for a weekly subscription to one of the intra-mural clubs. (The present-day equivalent of one shilling, or twelve old pence, is about £1.50.)

* 1931

There was no doubt that the members felt the Centre was their own club and that its existence and health depended on themselves. Perhaps their partial financial responsibility contributed to the feeling.

John Comerford made the Centre's acquaintance with his wife and children soon after it reopened in 1946. He wrote a book about his experiences of it.

> What I very soon noticed about the Peckham Centre was the genuine sense of ownership, as much as membership, which the people had. They speak naturally in the so-called editorial 'we'. This is simply because they have a strong sense of community and of creation. It is they, as much as the scientists themselves, who made and make the place a going concern. Of this they are aware. 'We soon found', they will tell you, 'that such-and-such wouldn't work – so we changed it to this.'*

Certainly, there was a marked absence of a 'them and us' attitude.

The assumption of responsibility for the Centre by nearly every member, both adult and child, was a measure of the Peckham Biologists' success in creating circumstances in which a sense of responsibility could develop. These circumstances formed a complex whole which is not easy to analyse. In this chapter, I have described a few important elements of the whole which had evolved by the time I came to know the Centre well. Some, like the design of the building and the family and local membership, arose out of the philosophy and insight that Scott Williamson brought to the inception of the Centre. The Biologists' attitude, as exemplified by the account of the enrolment talk quoted above, played an essential part. A contributory circumstance (as we shall see later) was the fact that every member of the family, however young, had – his parents permitting – the run of the whole building (the consultation block excepted), and was free to choose his occupation for himself from among a variety of the kinds of activities that children value, including what elsewhere in the case of children might have been considered 'doing nothing', that is wandering around and watching, sitting and dreaming, or chatting with friends. This situation arose out of the implementation of the last of the five essential conditions of the experiment that I listed at the beginning of this chapter. This crucial fifth condition which I shall try to describe in the next chapter, was what Scott Williamson called the freedom of the individual *and* his environment – in other words, the freedom of *everybody*. This condition required constant vigilance and, at the outset, faith and courage to maintain.

* 1947

Chapter 3

A Fifth Condition: A Sort of Anarchy

That health involves the ability to direct the course of one's own life had long been Scott Williamson's opinion, but it was not until some months after the opening of the main experiment (the St Mary's Road Centre) that he realised how far it was necessary to go in providing opportunity for the exercise of self-direction.

I H Pearse and G Scott Williamson published *The Case for Action* in 1931 after they had closed the preliminary experiment and were planning the main one. In it they wrote:

> Those engaging in each activity will be formed into a series of intramural clubs; for example, the swimming club, the chess club etc. Into these intramural clubs, each individual, subject to his inclinations and needs will be drafted by medical prescription at the time of or subsequent to his medical overhaul. Within each club, graded and balanced teams will measure their skill and progress with one another. Thus, for example, in the gymnasium during the evenings and on holidays, the members of the gymnasium club will meet in batches to carry on the exercises desired by each member and prescribed for each by the doctor at the medical overhaul... In the afternoon, the gymnasium will be used by the school-children, again according to the prescription given by the doctor.

How the authors must have chuckled if, when the new Centre was well under way, they had returned to the book they had written a few years earlier and read this passage, for the reality was so completely different. In their report of the first eighteen months of the St Mary's Road Centre, *Biologists in Search of Material*, they wrote:

> Our failures during our first eighteen months' work have taught us something very significant. Individuals, from infants to old people, resent or fail to show any interest in anything initially presented to them through discipline, regulation or instruction which is another aspect of authority.
>
> We now proceed by merely providing an environment rich in instruments for action – that is giving a chance to do things. Slowly but surely these chances are seized upon and used as opportunity for development of inherent capacity. The instruments of action have one common characteristic – they must speak for themselves.
>
> Having provided the members with a chance to do things, we find that we have to leave them to make their own use of them. We have had to learn to sit back and wait for these activities to emerge. Any

impatience on our part, translated into help, has strangled their efforts – we have had to cultivate more and more patience in ourselves. The alternative to this cultivation of patience is, of course, obvious – the application of compulsion in one or other of its many forms, perhaps the most tempting of which is persuasion. But having a fundamental interest in the source and origin of spontaneous action – as all biologists must – we have had to discard even that instrument for initiating activities.*

Their 'guinea pigs', as the members called themselves, were reminding them of the importance of meticulous adherence to the principles of research into health which, as Williamson and Pearse had themselves stated, stipulate the freedom of the object under study.

> ... any imposed action or activity becomes a study of authority, discipline or instruction and not the study of free agents plus their self-created environment.†

So, in order to be good scientists, they were forced to deny any desire they had to teach and lead the members of the Centre. It must have been hard, particularly if the experience of one's entire working life had convinced one of the importance for health of certain actions and behaviours. Indeed, it must have seemed like a dereliction of duty not to try to propel people gently along the road to physical fitness. But the sedentary frequenter of the cafeteria, the – apparently – confirmed spectator and the Whist addict were left in peace.

By the time I came to work at the Centre, sixteen months after it opened, it was evident to me that every member – child or adult – felt entirely free to choose his occupation, free too to do nothing; for a person is not free if he feels obliged to be engaged in activity.

> Dealing with matter or form, as the chemist does, with motion or force as the physicist does, or with isolated organs as the physiologists do, permits of a straightforward technique for conditioning and controlling the experiment. The biologists studying the human organism must deal with *free* agents...
>
> As one of our colleagues remarked – It seems that a 'sort of anarchy' is the first condition in any experiment in human applied biology. This condition is also that to which our members most readily respond...
>
> Within eighteen months, the seeming chaos and disorder is rapidly developing into something very different.
>
> So it would seem that a very strict 'anarchy', if we can use that term, will permit the emergence of order through spontaneous action, and so provide a field of observation for the biologist.¶

(According to the *Shorter Oxford English Dictionary*, the Greek derivation of the word 'anarchy' means 'no rule'.)

The patience of the Biologists was usually rewarded in time. Gradually, the spectators became also doers. It is probable, however, that some

---

* 1938, p. 38
† *ibid.*, p. 40
¶ *ibid.*, pp. 39–41

of the people who signed on as members were never tempted by the opportunity to extend their horizons to more varied experience, and eventually went elsewhere for their beer or whist, and that there were some who quietly disappeared because they were too shy to strike out on their own and too self-conscious to sit around watching others until the urge to join in came at last.

The children were far less inhibited. From the beginning crowds of them invaded the Centre every day after school was over. And they quickly sized up the situation: no-one was going to throw you out or even tell you off; you could do what you liked and go where you liked – just like a grown-up. But they were frustrated because debarred from where they most wanted to be – the gymnasium and the swimming pool, unless in the charge of an adult. For the first nine months, they made thorough nuisances of themselves and there was some minor vandalism. I know from experience that large enclosed spaces invite a child to run, for it used to happen with one or two of our own five when, as a family, we visited the British Museum or an ancient cathedral, so I am not surprised that the Peckham children spent their time racing along the gallery-like halls and up and down the stairs of a building that had been especially designed to facilitate the easy flow of people around it, only pausing to gaze longingly into the swimming pool and gymnasium, or that they shunted the heavy sliding window panels back and forth and played at curling with the solid glass cubes of ashtrays on the polished cork floor of the Long Room.

Nearly everyone begged Scott Williamson to do something about it – to exert his authority. But as he wrote in a letter to his sister at this time*:

> Our discoveries – if they are discoveries – point to *responsibility* as the biological characteristic of organism. Authority and responsibility are mutually antipathetic and, indeed, as they grow strong and adult, they are antagonistic.

Yet something other than patience seemed to be required to solve the problem of the children.

It was at this point, when the Centre had been open for about five months, that Lucy Crocker joined the staff. She gave up a promising career as a biology teacher and took a considerable drop in salary in order to do so. Later, for an appendix to Dr Pearce's book *The Quality of Life*, Lucy wrote the following account of how the problem of the children's use of the Centre was solved:

Only Look – The Answer is There

With so much to offer that appeals to children – a swimming bath, a gymnasium, a theatre – we started by assuming that they would be glad to make use of all this in the conventional way in groups with instructors,

---

* See *The Quality of Life*, p. 27

which was then the only way we knew. So we set about getting out timetables of activities.

Walking round the building we contacted the children. A gang chasing up the stairs engaged in some mysterious game would readily stop and talk. Yes, they would like gym classes. Oh yes, they would love to learn to swim, were keen on roller skates. We got their names and ages and we grouped them, girls and boys, seven to nine years, ten to thirteen, fourteen to sixteen, and we fixed times when they said they were free to come. We made sure that the gym and the bath were free and instructors available and we posted up lists for all to see. We thought that that was all that was needed in the way of initial effort, that from then on it would be a question of keeping things running. Little did we know!

For this is what happened. Although the whole timetable had been drawn up with the children's wholehearted co-operation, when the week came for the classes to start, only the odd child came. The others might appear in the building before the time of the class, or later that day – haring round as usual – and they seemed unable to give any precise reason why they had not turned up. By the end of the first week it was clear that they were not coming.

So we had to think again; on the brink of what was to be a long, laborious piece of original research, involving ever fresh thinking in terms of education and of biology before we had it clear. At this point I asked the Director if he minded how slowly I moved with the children, if he would give me six months? He said he did not mind how slowly I moved as long as I did move and not stand still.

Then started what seemed a long period of misery, for what we did was to walk round and round and up and down the building, watching the destruction, harassed by every well-wisher saying 'Can't you do something to stop the children breaking everything up?' The answer was that of course we could, but at the risk of driving them out.

But as we walked we watched, until we began to understand. The children came into the building, not as they went to school, that is because they had to, but because they liked to come and felt that they were entitled to (their parents paid!). They came to do what they liked and to enjoy themselves. It seemed that here in their free time even a swimming bath lacked appeal if its use involved instruction – though the instructors, as people, were well enough liked by them. Also, we saw that the times when they could come were often unpredictable and cut into by a host of duties – shopping, homework, music lessons, accompanying brothers and sisters – many more obligations than we had realised. Many things might arise at home or at school to prevent their coming at a given time.

At the same time there were signs that doing what they wanted to do was not altogether at variance with what was offered. The swimming bath tempted, the gymnasium with its ropes tempted, the open forum with skates and bicycles tempted. But somehow there was a barrier between these streaming children and the surrounding opportunities that they found themselves unable to surmount.

At last we saw the answer. The children must be admitted to the various activities individually, so let them get on with it.

One problem was that the two most attractive places had had to remain out of bounds because they were potentially so dangerous that no-one could take the responsibility of letting unsupervised children into them. If the children could play at curling in the long room where there was nothing but tables, chairs and ashtrays, what would they not do in the lofty gym thick with hanging ropes, rope ladders, poles, vaulting horses? Or the swimming bath – whenever you came into the building there it was, its green-blue water lapping as the eddies from some swimmer reached the edges. But it was dangerously deep at one end; who would dare let the inexperienced in to drown?

But some of the children could swim and this was easy to check: the swimming instructor could watch to see if the claim was true. If a child could swim the length would he not be safe? Then, let any child who can swim a length go into the bath for half an hour at any time he or she likes during the time that children of that age are allowed in the building unaccompanied by their parents. Once arrived at, the solution seems simple and obvious, especially now so many years later; but it must be remembered that at that time educationalists were all thinking in terms of classes and groups.

The technical problem was this: children, only some of whom could swim, were coming into the building all at different times. How could we control entry into the swimming bath in this circulating hubbub? There was already a check-point into the bath changing-rooms because adults paid to go in, but clearly a member of staff could not accompany each child there to give permission. A child would come tearing up to you in the billiard room, in the laboratory where you might be taking visitors round, out on the concrete where you were on your knees helping a six-year-old to lace up skate boots. So we took a piece of paper, scribbled the child's name, 'swimming' and our name, and off the child rushed to the man at the gate of the baths – and in about a minute he was 'in'. He had permission from a member of staff who knew him and knew that he could swim.

This permissive piece of paper proved the working clue to the whole problem of the children's use of the Centre. The next four years were spent by us in elaborating the technique, and by the children in ever more varied response to what we came to see as a challenge to them for the development of skill. About eighteen months after the Centre opened there were at last signs of order: not the quietness due to external discipline but the hum of active children going about their own business. The 'ticket system' as it developed is described on p. 197 of *The Peckham Experiment*, where we see that the 'ticket' came to be a common symbol current in the daily business of child and bionomist–curator alike, and equally essential to both for their business in the Centre.

By the time the 'ticket system' had become fully operational, up to 250 children were using the Centre every day, yet the only supervisory staff found to be necessary was the Curator of the Instruments of Health and one or at the most two student–assistants. By this time, the only professional instructor employed was a part-time woman swimming and keep-fit teacher. She spent most of her time teaching adults, for few could swim when they joined and her lessons were much sought after. Some children asked her help from time to time but, as she only taught the breast stroke, most preferred to teach themselves, progressing through 'dog-paddle' or a kind of overarm lunge to something resembling the crawl. Whether they were taught by her or taught themselves, they made swift progress because they concentrated hard on learning in order to be allowed the freedom of the 'big' pool.

There were many other activities open to the children that were eagerly taken up. Alongside the two full-size billiards tables there was a junior table and down in the 'office' there were cues and balls for the children to borrow. The badminton court, the table-tennis tables and the theatre stage were normally being used by adults, but, during the slack time for adults, between about 6pm and 8pm, the children were able to use them. Few adults wished to use the gymnasium and the children found it a very desirable playground. Long before the era of 'adventure playgrounds', there was 'free-play' in the Centre gymnasium. It came about in the following manner. Soon after the Centre opened, a young physical education teacher called Adelaide Crighton joined the staff. She waited in the gymnasium at the appointed times to teach the children who had opted for gymnastics classes. As Lucy Crocker has related, few children turned up, and Adelaide realised that even these were very lukewarm about being taught. So she introduced them to a game called 'Shipwrecks' (a similar game to 'Off ground'). All the apparatus, which was of a kind used in all well-equipped gymnasiums of the period, was got out and placed so that it was possible to move from piece to piece without once stepping on the floor. One child was 'catcher', if you were caught you became the catcher and all those 'drowned' because they touched the ground were 'out'. The children loved this game but did not like to be 'out', so Adelaide waived the rule; and the game went on and on and on. Day after day, it was all they wanted to do in the gym. By the time, in the autumn of 1936, when Adelaide left to return to her home in Canada, it was found unnecessary to have anyone minding the children as they played. At times they played shipwrecks, trying out new movements – monkey-like leaps and swings – as they played, but mostly they worked individually at devising new skills and actions, being 'Tarzan' or 'Jane'. They practised these acrobatic skills hour after hour and day after day, placing the movable equipment to suit their needs.

Some of the equipment was used in a way for which it was not intended and which horrified conventional teachers of gymnastics: knots were tied at the ends of the climbing ropes, for example, which after a time could never be untied. The play will be described in greater detail below and also some fascinating conjectures as to what motivated the children to behave in this way.

The curator looked down into the gym from time to time through the 'viewing window' in the Long Room on the first floor; and she controlled the entry to the gym by means of the 'tickets'. She divided the afternoon into two, reserving the earlier half, from 4pm to 5pm for the younger or less experienced and less confident children.

A child was required to obtain a ticket, not only in order to gain access to the pool and the gymnasium, but also to use any of the equipment that was available for the children's use.

Lucy Crocker designed cabinets and racks to hold the equipment, after it had been discovered which kinds of equipment, toys and games were most in demand. Her intention was to provide each object with its own appropriately shaped pigeon hole or niche. For example:

> ... the 36 pairs of booted roller skates of different sizes stand ranged in their appropriate pigeon holes, each hole labelled with the size of boot. The child finds his own size skates, takes them and deposits the ticket and his own shoes in the vacant hole. When each child finishes skating he takes his own shoes out of the pigeon hole, returns the skates and puts the ticket in the box placed for the purpose. Each bicycle, scooter, shinty stick and puck, racquet, book, jig-saw puzzle, game of draughts, chess or dominoes, each billiard cue and ball, sewing and drawing materials, an old typewriter etc etc, is in its own properly designed niche.*

These cabinets stood on castors and could easily be moved or locked up and temporarily withdrawn from use. Although the children were very rarely reminded to return the objects when they had finished with them to their places in the cabinets, they nearly always did so. It was as Lucy Crocker had guessed it might be: the fact that each object borrowed had a special place of its own into which it neatly fitted made an impression on the child which caused him[†] to want to round off his action by returning the object to its place. At the end of the day, the used tickets were collected from the boxes in which they had been accumulating so that a record could be made of the activity of each child.

The Curator, assisted by a student, saw to it that the equipment used by the children was in good repair and was available when required. A student was stationed by the store of roller skates, scooters, small bicycles and other equipment used on the partly covered outdoor playground and in the cricket practice nets. The Curator moved around the building observing what was going on. She was also responsible for booking out space or equipment to adults, and she made it her business, as far as possible, to become acquainted with every family. Therefore she might be engaged in conversation anywhere where she had a view into the swimming pool (no attendant was employed to stand inside the

* 1943, p. 197
† I have occasionally used 'he' to mean a child or adult of either sex.

glass-walled pool chamber); but she never stayed long in one place, for she kept herself continuously informed about what was going on in the gymnasium and the badminton court by looking down into them through the viewing windows in the walls of the Long Room. She carried with her a bundle of 'tickets', a different colour for each day, and the children would have to find her in order to get one.

Scott Williamson wanted to extend to the children the same opportunities for responsible and spontaneous action that he was trying to make possible for the adults. But he had not realised quite how selective they would in fact turn out to be. They proved to need to choose what to do from minute to minute – not days or weeks in advance.

As I shall describe later, during their play in the gymnasium, outdoor playground and pool, they made the most of the opportunity to choose, not just from minute to minute but from second to second or fraction of a second, where and how to move. They not only selected an activity, but also, while engaged in this activity, continuously exercised choice of action. But the words 'choose' or 'select' imply deliberation, so neither is right to describe their behaviour. They were continually responding to the changing circumstances of their surroundings and, at the same time, to their own learning-needs.

Responsibility went with this spontaneity it appeared – responsibility for themselves, and for their surroundings: within a year of Lucy Crocker's appointment, the behaviour of the children had completely changed. From being utter nuisances, they became a pleasure to have around. As a result, the adults' attitude to them changed and this in turn increased the children's self-respect and respect for the adults.

Visitors to the Centre began to remark on the purposeful air of the children as they moved around the building, on their serenity and poise and the direct and friendly way in which they responded to a stranger's questions.

As the adults began to group together to pursue activities, Scott Williamson found that vigilance was necessary to ensure that *everybody* was free to exercise their faculties and develop their talents. It was necessary to guard against the possibility of established groups inadvertently monopolising the available space, and to ensure that those members with a talent for organisation did not exercise it to the extent of curtailing the autonomy or inhibiting the spontaneity of others. The history of the billiards club provides an example of the way in which the Biologists acted.

Two billiards tables and a junior one were some of the few pieces of equipment installed at the opening. Very soon there was a flourishing billiards club. They installed a cupboard in which they could lock up cues and balls and proceeded to occupy both tables all and every evening. Scott Williamson, together with Jack Donaldson who was at that time on

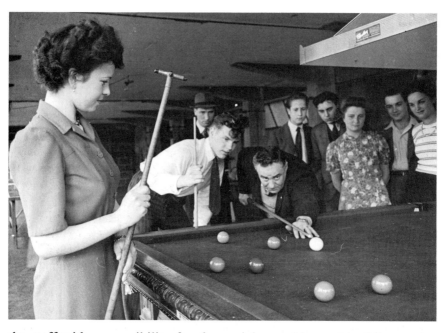

the staff with responsibility for the social amenities and building maintenance, arranged a meeting with the club and explained the situation to
them. It was agreed that one of the large tables and the small one would
be at all times left free for the use of people who did not belong to the
billiards club. This arrangement continued to work well throughout the
existence of the Centre. Almost always there was a member of the club
playing and the billiards club were glad of the opportunity it gave them
to spot and recruit new talent for the club. He would lend the club's cues
and balls to anyone wanting to use the non-club table. Otherwise a key
of the cupboard where the club's cues and balls were kept could be
obtained from the office off the cafeteria. The club members made
themselves responsible for the care and upkeep of the tables and no-one
can remember any damage.

As clubs and societies of enthusiasts for particular activities formed,
the Curator of the Instruments for Health took care that space was
always available for new initiatives and that the casual user, the diffident
beginner and the children and adolescents were never crowded out. For
instance, the water polo club was allotted the 9.30pm to 10pm period for
their games. For the rest of the evening the pool was free for family and
general swimming.

There was some competition for the use of the theatre/badminton
court between the badminton players and the various groups that formed
from time to time to produce plays, reviews and operettas. Badminton
was so popular that it might have become necessary eventually for the

keenest and most expert players to join an outside badminton club in order to get the number of games they desired, and to leave the court free for newcomers and the more casual players, and the theatre free half the time for rehearsals of plays etc.

The limitation on the freedom of staff and members to organise others, except at their request and for a limited period, and the restriction of rules and regulations was maintained at the Centre by an ultimate authority in the person of Dr Scott Williamson, for he was the director of this most unusual research establishment. But he very rarely exercised any authority. He was often heard to say, 'I am the only person with authority and I use it only to prevent anybody from using authority over anybody else.'

'Don't make rules in order to make your job easier,' he told his assistants. It was almost the only directive he gave them. He left them to find their own way but pulled them up if they were straying from their role as scientists who, he said, must exercise 'the laboratory scientist's discipline which allows facts to speak for themselves' – very difficult to do, he conceded, because 'in human biology, the facts are actions.' Harold (Adge) Elven remembers being told, on one occasion after the war when he was a part-time member of the staff, 'Don't you ever put ideas into their heads. Just listen and report back to us.' Elsie Purser was also a part-time member of the staff after the war. She said that she often found herself reading a story to some of the younger schoolchildren when they came to the Centre after school was over. They would bring a book to her wherever she happened to be and sit down round her on the floor. 'I did not get a book myself and say, would you like a story? That would have got me into trouble with the Doctor.' At one stage, Lucy Crocker gave the gatekeeper instructions not to let unaccompanied children under a certain age (probably 13 or 14) enter the building after 8pm. Scott Williamson told her to rescind the order: she herself, he said, should contact the child and should judge each case on its merits. It was up to her to notice if children whom she considered too young or too irresponsible to be welcome to the other members were roaming the building after 8pm when the adult activities were in full swing, and to tell them to stay close to their parents or, if these were not in the building, to go home.

The quest for leaders – a fashionable sociological pursuit at the time – was not followed by the Biologists. They were hoping that life in the Centre would bring out the individuality, initiative and creativity in people so that there would be fewer and fewer sheep among them wanting to be led. This did in fact happen. The members welcomed the services of the individuals who had a talent, for instance, for producing plays or organising sing-songs, dance bands, parties and celebrations, or those with enthusiasms who were willing to pass on their skills and knowledge when requested, but they appeared to feel no obligation to reward them by institutionalising them. New talent and ideas, individual initiatives and leaders of new ventures were always emerging, but it was the followers who decided individually who they would follow and for how long. As time went on, fewer and fewer of the members were sheep waiting to be led and self-imposed leaders did not last long. So it became less and less necessary for Scott Williamson to take action to guard the freedom of all from any threat that an individual's talent for leadership or organisation might constitute. There was one member, an official of a printer's trade union, who would corner Dr Williamson from time to time and argue in favour of political democracy and majority rule within the Centre; he wanted a central organising committee of members, but he commanded no following. The Biologists wrote of the Centre, 'One of its outstanding characteristics is its fluidity which permits the growth and continuous evolution of its society from day to day and year to year.'*

Sociologists have criticised Scott Williamson on the grounds that his research subjects were self-selected. This was true, in that the Centre tended to attract and retain as members people who had not lost their potentiality for health. Some of the families, who disappeared without giving any reason, may have let their membership lapse after a short time because it worried them to be left to use their initiative; perhaps they wanted to be organised, shepherded and entertained. To some extent the Centre acted as a sieve in which people with a healthy urge to grow – to realise their potentiality, to develop their physical, mental and social talents and skills – were retained. Since the Peckham Biologists' aim was the study of health, this served them well. They had not set up their research station in order to study the activity of the average person in the normal situation to be found outside the Centre.

It is interesting to note that many families joined because the children had persuaded their parents to give it a try. Children would have heard about it from schoolmates or watched, from the road, the roller skating on the forecourt, or they might have been invited in to see what went on by the parents of their friends who were members, and then nagged their own parents for as long as was necessary.

In the afternoon nurseries for under-fives, the children took to freedom and self-regulation like ducks to water. The nurseries and their equipment were very carefully designed to suit the desires and needs of babies and toddlers for activity. The polished cork-covered floors offered a warm and resilient surface on which to creep and crawl and run barefoot. In the babies' nursery, besides the more usual toys, there was a short railed-in slide and steps which was much used by babies long before they could walk. They crawled up the steps and slid down the short slide to the polished floor on their tummies, or bottoms or pulled

* 1943

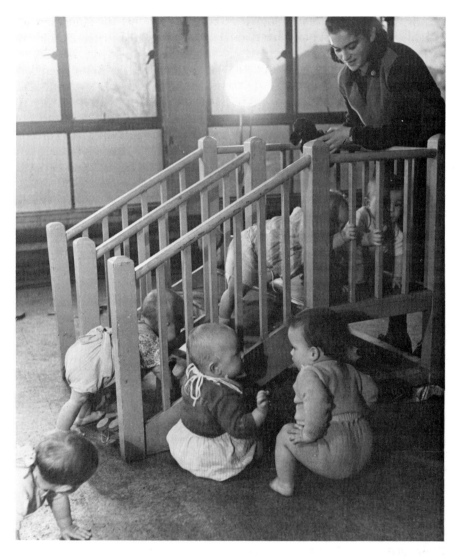

themselves up the steps and down again holding on to the rails, or hauled themselves up the slope and bumped down the steps. On the tables (or the floor, according to the age of the baby) were placed cots, designed by Dr Pearse. These 'box hammocks' consisted of four boards about six or seven inches wide standing on their sides forming a rectangle and acting as the sides and legs of the cot with a piece of canvas filling in the rectangle about half way up the sides. The babies could crawl or roll out of these cots when they felt ready for more movement. Even earlier they could raise their heads as they lay in them and see around, identifying noises and matching sights to sounds.

The babies and children in the Centre nurseries did not lack stimulation. They received plenty from the activity of the other children, some of whom were likely to be either older, more active in temperament, or more advanced due to having had the stimulating presence of older brothers or sisters at home. But these environmental happenings did not force themselves on the attention of the babies, who were free to choose to what they would attend. When an adult does the stimulating, the situation is quite different, for an adult tends to claim the small child's attention, so that he is not free to direct it where he will, and if he is not interested in or attracted to what the adult offers, he may have to take the negative path of shutting off his attention and retiring into himself.

Of course babies need adults. It may be that up to the age of about six months, they need to be continuously in contact with the body of one.* Later they need models of various ages on which to exercise their instinct to imitate. But they also need opportunity to exercise their potential faculty to choose, for themselves and from moment to moment, the experiences and activities they need for the development of their mental and physical capabilities. The faculty to recognise what one needs to do for the growth of one's abilities is like any other faculty; it requires exercise if it is to develop. (More of this later in the book.) In the Centre nurseries there was no superfluity of staff with idle hands looking for opportunities to exercise *their* faculties *on* the children and, in the process, unwittingly depriving them of the chance for adventure and learning.

The Peckham Biologists tried to find out what kind of physical surroundings give children of nursery and pre-school age the opportunity for the sort of activity they desire. As with the older children, they found that the more successful one is in providing such surroundings the less one needs to organise, entertain, teach or play with the children. When left to themselves in a suitable environment, they are constantly physically and mentally – or just mentally – active.

But they do need watching at this age. When they realise that the adult in charge is not going to intervene at every moment to save them from the effects of their own and others' actions, they will take the responsibility for their own safety and enjoyment – however young. But they can only be as responsible as their knowledge of things and people allows. One must plan and arrange the surroundings to suit the likely knowledge of the age group and one must unobtrusively watch. For there may always be one child in a group who tends to be a bit reckless or at least over ambitious, or impatient of others getting in his way, or is – to an adult – unbelievably ignorant of the fact that the other children feel pain when hit or bitten. So one needs to be on one's toes. And yet it is rarely necessary to intervene, restrain or help, as I discovered when I ran a playgroup for twelve children aged two to five single handed.

* See Liedloff 1974, and Chapter 9 below

I had little chance to observe the behaviour of the children in the Centre nurseries for, apart from taking the more competent three and four year olds into the gymnasium and the learners' swimming pool during the early afternoons before the schoolchildren arrived, my job was to help to make the play facilities available to the latter. My knowledge of the behaviour of very young children in a free-play situation, where only the physical environment – not the children – is organised, was obtained mainly during the fourteen years I ran a playgroup on Peckham lines in my own house and garden, some years later.*

I was neither trained to teach nor keen on organising people, so while supervising this playgroup, I found it easy to fade into the background, and, being on my own, I was not distracted from watching.

I observed that, on joining the group, many of the children spent some days or weeks mostly watching the others. Sometimes this worried a parent, who felt the child was unhappy. But usually one could see, from the changing expressions on their faces, that they were totally absorbed and interested in what they saw and heard and were far from being unhappy or frustrated. Incidentally, I observed that children who pondered a little before acting often became skilled more quickly than those who rushed in impulsively; for the latter tended to be inept at first, making unnecessary and inappropriate movements that became habits which had subsequently to be unlearned, if the child was to obtain a degree of skill that satisfied him.

A few children talked incessantly as they played; a few were almost entirely silent for months on end, although quite talkative at home.

Most seemed to be well aware of what the other children were doing, for conversations went on across the room, and, even when running, jumping or sliding down a plank among others painting, playing with bricks and many other things in a room 15 feet square, they did not get in each other's way (except, occasionally, on purpose, in order to tease).

It is impossible to act effectively or appropriately in a totally strange or constantly changing environment. For this reason among others I kept the fee per session low and most children attended every available session (five mornings a week at one period, later three), so they knew each other well. Also I took pains to keep the basic arrangement of the equipment in the playroom and in the garden the same from day to day. Therefore it was easy for them to make themselves familiar with their environment, both material and human. A newcomer's name was quickly learned although they were not formally introduced to each other. There were sympathies and antipathies, but rarely was any criticism expressed by one child of another: individualities, including (in that area at the time) the only very occasional black skin, and even weird eccentricities, were accepted without comment. It seems that, since to children of this age (mostly under four) all life is new, they expect variety. They never

* This playgroup is described in detail in *The Self Respecting Child*, Stallibrass, 1974

expressed criticism of others' skill except perhaps if it spoilt a game, and even then they were resilient, and made little fuss. New games and 'tricks' on the climbing and other apparatus were always being invented and some of these became traditional – passed on from one 'generation' to the next, like children's 'street games'.

I found that, if plenty of the most popular equipment was at all times available, squabbles were few and far between. One could observe a child occupying himself with something that was evidently a second choice because he would then leave it like a flash for some toy or piece of equipment that another child had just left. Here I must explain that I had found it necessary to make it known that I did not condone the use of superior strength of muscle or personality to relieve another child of a toy or piece of equipment. I did this by stepping in whenever it occurred and insisting on restitution. This behaviour on my part soon had an effect, because, I think, there was so much that the children wanted passionately to do that they avoided putting themselves into a position where they would have to do anything that would waste their time such as being made to restore the piece of equipment to its former user. So it soon became the custom that only if a child left a toy or a piece of apparatus was it available to another.

It seems that in this kind of playgroup, children learn to exercise self-control with ease. Perhaps it comes easily because they are incessantly practising control over their limbs and muscles, and this is easily extended to include their behaviour as a whole. Certainly it is evident that they restrain their impulses if they feel it is necessary for the preservation of the play situation they have chosen or are creating. In fact, their spontaneity never consists only of acting on impulse, for they take reality into account: they tend to attempt only those things that their own capacity and the facts of their present environmental situation make possible, and they do what fits into the whole formed by the activity of all the others.

The children were intent on their chosen learning-activities, which included learning about other children. It was very apparent that these children – both girls and boys – were very interested in people. Most of them were obviously enjoying the experience of learning how to play harmoniously and creatively with other children.

All in all, they were following the 'categorical imperatives' of childhood: developing their human and individual faculties to the limits of their potentiality and making themselves well acquainted with the world – with things and people, in order to become more and more effective and capable. On analysing their activity, one is astounded to realise how many different kinds of knowledge and skill these children were acquiring simultaneously. Many played solitary or communal make-believe games *at the same time as* they climbed or swung or jumped from the climbing frames or the apple tree, climbed up or slid down the slides or lino-covered bank, poured water, dug in the sand, rode scooters or bicycles or pushed prams and trolleys. They combined the two kinds of play, the two kinds of learning-activity.

I think what happened in my playgroup demonstrates how order, harmony and creativity can and do emerge in conditions of 'strict anarchy'.

This phenomenon was even more clearly observable in the Centre gym. Here a spectator could hardly avoid seeing that the children were individually aware at every moment of the total situation in the hall full of moving bodies and were fitting their movements into it. The gym was conventionally equipped, with ropes and rope ladders suspended from a ceiling two storeys high, wall bars along two walls, a 'window frame' reaching almost to the ceiling and covering one end wall. There were booms, vaulting bucks, balancing forms, parallel bars, a punch ball, coconut matting and so on and an ingeniously sprung cork-covered floor*. For the sake of the floor and to enable the children to use their toes for balancing and gripping and to become sure-footed, a barefoot rule was rigorously enforced.

There were sometimes as many as 30 children in the gym at one time but no instructor. The children would be running after each other (perhaps playing 'Off ground') sliding down the balancing forms, jumping from everywhere, swinging on the ropes, playing with balls, doing handsprings or wrestling. One of the favourite activities was to swing on a rope between the wall bars and a vaulting buck (or between two bucks) that they had positioned so that they could land neatly upon them. To do this successfully required very accurately timed and co-ordinated movement and the exercise of sensory judgement, and yet skill in this particular activity was not confined to a few gifted individuals. The ropes were constantly being used for this purpose, much more rarely for climbing. More recently, I watched some boys and girls including adolescents enjoying an exactly similar activity in the Playpark in Battersea Park, London. They had a long rope suspended from the limb of a very tall tree and they were leaping on to the swinging rope from the top of a high platform they had constructed with the help of the playleader.

With all this varied activity going on simultaneously in the Centre gym, there were no collisions. The children not only exercised judgement in moving in relation to the apparatus, but also in moving in relation to the movements of the other children, for they threaded their way with accuracy and speed among their constantly moving companions. Although each was obviously intent on his own purpose, he was apparently also aware of what all the children in his vicinity were doing and of what they were likely to do in the next fraction of a second.

* Described in Chapter 2

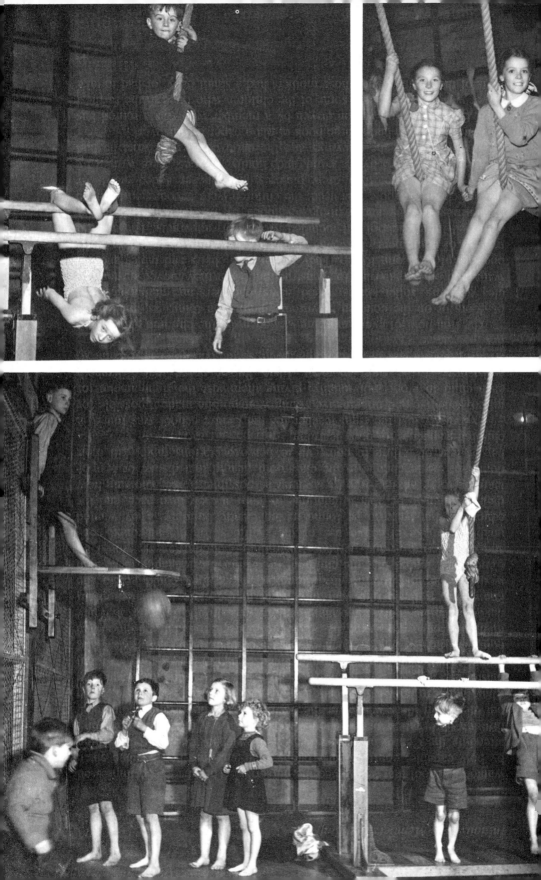

The scene could be terrifying to an adult at first glance, probably because no group of adults could have done what these children were doing. If the gym had contained adults instead of children, there would have been no activity except for false starts, apologies and 'after you's. Yet, judging from the popularity of the free-gym, these average and ordinary children were eager to practise the constant awareness and split-second decision-making that was required in order to weave their actions into the continuously changing three-dimensional pattern of the activity in the gym.

It was similar on the outdoor playground, where roller skating and the riding of small bicycles were the main activities, and also in the pool, where one rarely saw a child swimming 'lengths'. Instead they played, seemingly intent on discovering all the movements it is possible to make in and over a new element – water. I have watched children (mostly small boys) playing in a similar manner on a Saturday morning in a public pool. Everywhere, their intention seemed to be to acquire the ability to make their bodies obey them perfectly in the execution of a variety of movements and skills in the most challenging circumstances they could find. Evidently the presence of twenty or thirty spontaneously moving children increased the challenge, the hazards, the complexity of the situation, and, therefore, the degree of skill required – and the enjoyment.

As to the children's extraordinary ability to anticipate the situation during the next second or two, I wonder if the following circumstances helped to account for it. On the outdoor playground, for example, there was no rule or tradition (at least while I was there) causing everyone to skate or cycle in the same direction round the playground, but each of the more experienced children would know all there was to know about riding bicycles and skates, and what it is necessary to do in order to keep one's balance on them or to move in a desired direction. Each child would be aware of the practical restraints on the children's activity as well as of the potentialities of the sport, and this would make it easier for him to guess the likely direction and speed at any moment of the other child or children. The same sort of thing applied in the gym. The children had a purpose in common: the acquisition of agility, perfect balance and the sensory-motor control and co-ordination of the body as a whole. They were all absorbed in the same kind of learning-activity; their minds were on the same wavelength, as it were.

In the gym there was another factor: the main pieces of apparatus were either permanently fixed, or were positioned by the children them-selves, so it was easy for the children to be familiar with the physical geography of the hall. They were also familiar or becoming familiar with the properties and 'behaviour' of these inanimate objects. (An example of the behaviour of an object that children have to learn about sooner or

later is the pendulum action of a swing. This is something toddlers are
unlikely to know about and need to be guarded from as they often are by
means of a low rail in playgrounds.)

It is certain that the children could not have achieved the unremitting
concentration necessary for enjoyable play in these circumstances if they
had not been completely unselfconscious. In contrast, in a gymnastics
class when each child in turn is instructed to do a particular exercise on
a vaulting buck (the teacher hovering to catch him if he falls) and all the
others watch, one is, in effect, saying, in Pearse and Crocker's words,

> You give all your attention to what you are doing. We'll keep the rest of
> the world away. Be as egoistical as you like.*

In that situation 'egoism' is being cultivated, and the child's environment
is entirely passive. In the Centre gym, the environment was freely active.

Pearse and Crocker make the point that the children running, leaping
or swinging on the ends of ropes do not *avoid* each other; they swing or
run where there is (for a moment) space. A child does not focus on the
other children each in turn and aim to give way to each. Instead, he
looks for a space. At any moment, he might have a choice of spaces or
he might have to wait a few seconds. The child is being neither selfish
nor altruistic (putting someone's welfare before one's own). Instead, he
is fitting his activity into the whole formed by the activity of all the
children. In order to do this, he must be constantly aware of the total
situation in time and space in his vicinity. Therefore he cannot afford to
be distracted by extraneous thoughts such as, 'What are the onlookers up
there at the window thinking of me and my exploits? Am I leaping and
landing better than my pal? Am I doing it better than last time?' or, 'I
am ashamed to do it so badly.'

The children must have acquired and must hold, in their heads or –
more accurately – in their bodies, a great deal of information. This
includes:

> The nature and behaviour of the objects on which they climb.
> The nature of the medium (air or water) in which they move.
> The nature of the surface on or above which they move (water,
>   concrete, or sprung, cork-covered floor).
> The effects of the force of gravity on their bodies as they move.
> Their own present capabilities.
> The activity of the other children and the likely speed and direction of
>   their movements in the next fraction of a second.

Often, it was noticed, two or three children would be watching from
vantage points such as the top of the wall bars or of a rope ladder. I would
judge that, while 'resting', they were making mental notes of the inventions
of others for their own future use. But, down in the mêlée again, they were

* 1943, p. 192

obliged, like the little ones in my playgroup, to attempt to do only what it was possible to do, taking all the relevant factors into account. They were learning how to accommodate their desires and intentions to reality. They were exercising an easy self-control (one could call it spontaneous character-formation), together with an awareness of the needs of the whole. Each was, in effect, exercising responsibility for the smooth running and maintenance of the whole at the same time as he enriched it by his individual creativity. There was responsibility for the whole because one valued the whole – in this case, a rewarding play-situation.

When describing this kind of phenomenon, one tends to give the impression that the children were intellectually conscious of their needs and of the need to preserve the free-play amenity in gym and pool and that their behaviour was the result of reasoning. But it is probably true to say that most of the time the children were acting more as an organ of the body does when it acts for the good of the whole body on which it depends for existence and well-being. Certainly each child was, like a cell in a body, acting autonomously in Scott Williamson's sense of the word. He used autonomy not merely in the sense of self-government or self-direction but in the sense of spontaneously self-directed action in relation to the needs of the whole. (More about this in Chapter 10.)

Whether or not I am right in my explanation of what happened in the gym – and continued to happen over so many years – it was clear to anyone watching from the 'window' in the wall of the Long Room that the children did not make rules for themselves nor did some organise and direct the others, and yet order and harmony reigned.

There is another question to answer. Why did the children purposefully seek out this kind of play situation? Why did they demand this 'sort of anarchy'? Perhaps some light is thrown on the problem by the results obtained by Dr Harry Harlow in his experimental work with Rhesus monkeys. He reared a number of monkeys, keeping them in small cages, each with his mother or, in some cases, with three companions of the same age. He allowed some of them to spend 30 minutes a day in a playroom especially constructed to simulate the terrain in which young Rhesus would normally play. As Harlow said, these young monkeys developed 'a complex pattern of violent activity, performed with lightning speed and integrating all objects animate and inanimate in the room'.* At an age when Rhesus monkeys are normally able to fend successfully for themselves, these monkeys were released onto an island inhabited by wild Rhesus monkeys together with a group that had been reared similarly except that they had had no access to the playroom. The behaviour of the first group was soon indistinguishable from that of the wild monkeys, and they became assimilated into the colony. The second never did; they were 'socially incompetent', 'abnormally aggressive' and 'unable to mate successfully'.

* 1962

Were the Centre children, one wonders, instinctively seeking to acquire a skill that is – and always has been – important to human groups, the skill of being oneself and, at the same time, a part of a harmoniously effective social whole? Were they learning a basic kind of sociability – the art of fitting their own purposes into the whole formed by the activities of others?

In the Centre gym, it was not hard for a child to pursue his individual purpose and, at the same time, contribute to the diversity and harmony of the whole, as long as he was exercising an awareness of the total dynamic situation in his vicinity as well as a precise control of his movements in space and time. But one would have thought that, in the arena of the general social life of the Centre, it must have been very much harder, because of the varied nature of the activity, much of it as yet outside his experience and beyond his understanding. Yet, after the introduction of the 'ticket system' and free-play in the gym, pool and playground, the great majority of the children appeared to be doing just this. They moved among the adults in a serene and unobtrusive manner. Could this have come about partly because the children were able to generalise the skill described above which they had acquired in the predominantly physical situation of the gym etc, to the more varied and complex situation pertaining in the adult-orientated society of the Centre as a whole?

Whatever the cause, they became responsible and agreeable members of the society of the Centre, which was, of course, like that in the gym, one in which order had arisen in conditions – laid down and maintained by the Biologists – of 'strict anarchy'.

However, it was the free-gym that provided the most obvious example of the exercise of responsibility by the children. It showed that doing what you want to do, when what you want to do includes maintaining the existence and well-being of the whole on which you depend for enjoyment, can result in order, harmony and creativity.

My desire to explain thoroughly the essential fifth environmental condition that the Biologists laid down for their experiment has perhaps led me to a discussion of their central discoveries concerning health too early in the book. I shall continue now with the description of the operation of the Centre.

Chapter 4

Initiatives by Members and Staff

1. Intra-mural clubs

As I have told, the management made sure that there was always opportunity for spontaneous individual activity, but, in order to play a game or
exercise a skill with others on a regular basis, clubs were formed by
members. The badminton and billiards clubs have already been mentioned. There were, at most times throughout the Centre's existence,
boxing, fencing, radio, gramophone, photography, water polo, table tennis
and darts clubs. There were also groups who organised regular whist
drives, keep-fit and Women's League of Health and Beauty classes and
sometimes tap-dancing classes, as well as a 'Tuppeny Hop' every
Thursday evening in the Theatre, when the latest dance steps were
practised. Members would at times pass on their skills to other members
in first aid, woodwork, the playing of a musical instrument, choral
singing, diving or dressmaking. There was always a group preparing a
dramatic performance – a play, review, 'concert party' or operetta.

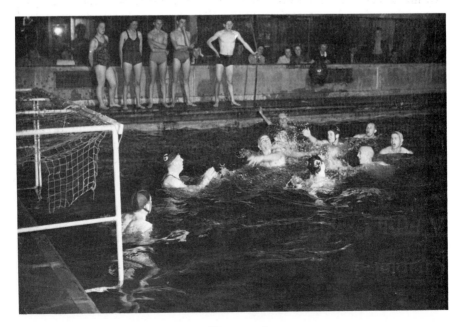

Water polo

The secretaries of these clubs and groups collected subscriptions from their members – three or six old pence per week, and paid a proportion of the money to the Centre as rent; the amount varying according to whether the club provided its own equipment or borrowed it from the Centre.

2. Ballroom dancing

Dancing was a very popular activity and very skilled. (It was the era of the Palais de Danse.) All ages took part, more women than men, but women danced quite happily together. The Long Room, its floor tiled with polished cork, made an ideal dance hall, with room for spectators and sitters-out in the aisles between the pillars.

During 1937 Lucy Crocker more than once asked some of the adolescent boys who were often seen watching the dancing with fascination (girls of the same age easily found partners) if they would like to have dancing classes arranged for them; but no, they would rather just watch a little when they felt like it. Then, it was noticed that some of these boys of 14 or 15 were practising in corners as much out of sight as they could get while remaining within the sound of the music. The next development was that they found a dancing enthusiast, a young man of 19 or 20 who was willing to teach them. They brought him to Lucy to book space for a weekly class and the loan of a gramophone and records. (One of these boys, Adge Elven, found himself, eight or nine years later, conducting dancing classes himself, as Mrs Purser tells.*) Soon, the instructor found himself overwhelmed by the number of pupils (girls as well as boys) and he divided the second-floor hall (above the Long

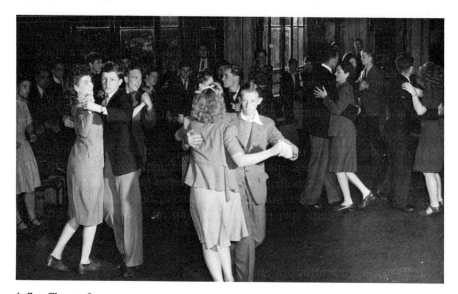

* See Chapter 8

Room) into sections by means of chairs and recruited young men and women from his dancing acquaintances to help teach.

3. The Centre dance band

Early in the pre-war years, a dance band was started by a Centre member who had formally been a member of the famous Ambrose's Dance Band. The centre band became extremely competent under his leadership, practising assiduously during the week in one of the secluded 'committee rooms' and playing regularly on Saturday evenings as well as for special occasions, up to the outbreak of war. After the war, two or three talented pianists played for dancing, and on Saturdays and special occasions a band would materialise and, at all times, dancers could rely on the radio club to relay gramophone records to the part of the building where dancing was to take place.

4. The Centre farm

In 1935, Dr Pearse rented Oakley House at Bromley Common, Kent (seven miles from Peckham). Several of the staff lodged in the house, and on the 77 acres round it a herd of Jersey cows was pastured and preparations were made to grow vegetables and fruit. The two doctors had found that the vegetables on sale in the Peckham shops were frequently stale and the milk was either pasteurised or unsafe. Tuberculin-tested milk was prohibitively expensive. Within a year of acquiring Oakley House, raw milk from the tuberculin-tested Jersey herd was on sale in the Centre at the current price of ordinary milk in the area. When the soil had begun to be revitalised by Sir Albert Howard's 'Indore' composting method of fertilising, vegetables and fruit grown on the farm were also sold in the cafeteria. Pregnant families and those with small children were given first option. Before the war 'Scofa' bread was used in the cafeteria. After the war all the bread was made by a local baker with stone ground flour from 100 per cent of the wheat grain.

When the Centre reopened in 1946, Oakley House and its grounds had to be retrieved from the Admiralty (who had had it from the RAF) and restocked. The first cow was bought with money subscribed by member-families on their own initiative.

5. Camping

In 1936, Captain Victor Cazalet MP lent an area of his estate at Sissinghurst in Kent to the Centre for a camping site. It included a wood surrounding a lake and a disused oast house.

Margaret Nash recalls:

A Camping Club was formed of which my father was Secretary and a band of members worked down there each weekend making it habitable for families to spend some time in the country. The two 'roundles' became 'ladies' and 'gents' dormitories and there was a communal room with tables, chairs, cupboards for food and several gas cooking hobs. Also through the woods was a lake where we could swim and there was a rowing boat too. We had lovely weekends there staying in the Oast House but for our two week holiday we took a large family tent and camped in style. We were lucky enough to have a car but others came on motor bikes, some with sidecars and others cycled all the way. In fact it was at the camp that John and I first met. He had cycled down with a couple who had a tandem, but being a bit of a 'loner' my mother felt sorry for him and took him under her wing and suggested he had his meals with us.

Captain Cazalet was killed during the war and, when the Centre reopened, the camp was no longer available. However, some families began to spend their Sundays at the Centre farm at Oakley House, which was easily reached by train and bus from Peckham. Soon a camping club had formed and space was found on the pastures for tents, which were stored, when not in use, with the members' other camping equipment in a large hut the RAF had built for a gymnasium, the exposed rafters being useful for hanging the tents up to dry. Twenty families might be camping there at a weekend, and during the school summer holidays, mothers would spend a month there with their children, while fathers came at weekends or, more often, commuted from the camp. 'We used to do work on the farm,' Harry Coring said. 'My son drove a tractor when he was ten, and the children used to watch the calves being born.'

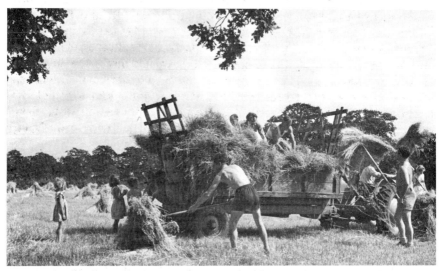

Helping with the harvest

6. War-time evacuation to Oakley House

Already, at the time of the Munich crisis, the Biologists had made plans to use Oakley House as a place to which member-families with young children could be evacuated in case of war. When war came, 29 families, including 50 children under five, chose to go there with a view to working the farm and providing themselves with good quality food. They chose to do this rather than to avail themselves of the government facilities and financial assistance for evacuation.

The warm and sunny weather in September 1939 was a great help in the settling-in period. When the fear of immediate enemy bombing of London had subsided, about one third of the families returned home. The rest stayed, and the mothers began to divide up the farm, garden and household work and the care of the children between them. Fortunately the Montessori Society had appointed two teachers to start an experimental school in the Centre in September, and wished to transfer the scheme to the farm. An adjoining cottage was adapted (by some fathers) for use as a school, and all the children who had mastered the art of walking spent the day there, or in the garden, from 8.30am to 5pm. In a pamphlet *War and the Family* (May 1940) Innes Pearse and Lucy Crocker wrote:

> The teachers receive a good deal of help from some of the mothers; and the children, during the time they were out of doors, mingled freely with the mothers working on the farm. In fine weather, mothers of young babies brought them in their prams into the vegetable garden to be near them while they worked.

A horticulturalist, Dorothy Coupe, who had been at one time a member of the staff of the Pioneer Health Centre, took over the direction of the farm and the large walled vegetable garden, and the receptionist at the Centre, the invincible Amy Moor, the household. As long as the original farm workers remained, the mothers were able to get some help and instruction from them, but, within a month or two, they were doing all the work themselves, except for help at weekends from some of the fathers still working in London. They and the husbands on leave from the forces did most of the wood chopping, digging, electrical work and plumbing.

Mrs Ethelyn Hazell was one of the mothers. She recalled:

> The women were divided into groups of four or five and changed jobs weekly, gardening, cooking and housework for instance. Some were lazy and didn't want to pull their weight. This was a bit of a problem because the co-operation of all was necessary for the success of the scheme. We fed ourselves from the market garden and the farm. The scheme was an unusual undertaking, since it provided the means of keeping families together and made it possible for women with small children still to make a contribution to the war effort. The Ministries of Health and

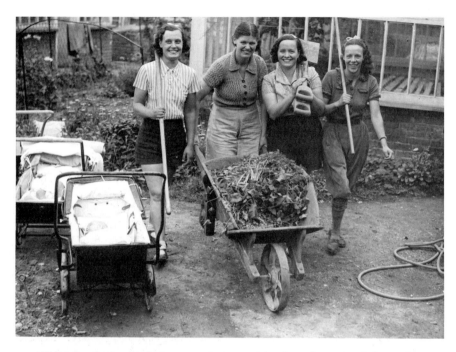

Education began by being very interested in the scheme, and for a short time we even enjoyed the title of MAYS (Mothers' Auxiliary Yeoman Service). However, after one long night preparing full accounts and details of the scheme for the expected visit the following morning of the two Ministries concerned, we were informed that they were no longer interested in anything other than mothers going into factories and children going elsewhere.

I acted as typist and 'orderly' at first. And then, not without misgivings because I was afraid of cows, I volunteered to help with milk production. I hoped I would be able to work in the dairy, but I found I was a natural milker and loved the Jersey cows and all the work involved. When the herdsman was called up, I took on his job with one assistant. Cows get used to people and prefer to be milked and herded by the same person every day. We were trained by an instructor from the Agricultural College at Wye in Kent which was closed at the time.

Part of my job was to help with the material from the cowsheds, kale fields etc. for our compost heaps, subsequently used in the gardens and farm. Everything was grown organically. The Centre Doctors saw clearly the need for study of the evidence concerning soil fertility and health and, with Lady Eve Balfour and others formed the Haughley Trust in 1939 and, later, the Soil Association.

It was a pity we had to leave after a year because we all benefitted enormously. We learned new skills, and some people became really interested in the farm and garden work. Some had never done any gardening or fruit picking etc. before. Mothers who had been suffering from some minor ailment improved in health. In our turn in the kitchen, we learned about the cooking of home and naturally grown vegetables. We did get a revolt when Dr Pearse tried to insist on the children having only wholewheat porridge for their breakfast which they took in the communal dining room with their mothers – and fathers when they visited. Many of them were used to every imaginable kind of packetted cereal. The children slept in two big rooms together, with one mother on duty, and we mothers slept in dormitories. A few small bedrooms were 'married quarters' which could be booked in advance for a night or a weekend.

At the end of nine months, in spite of the absence of enemy action over Britain, there were twelve mothers still at the farm. They had survived an exceptionally long cold winter, and had overcome their town-dwellers' fear of animals and dislike of what they thought of as 'dirt'; they had adjusted to living in a very cold house with the minimum of comfort and to communal living. The seven or eight who had previously returned home had felt it was better to be looking after their husbands and their own homes, but most had gone with regret, for they had been long enough on the farm for its good effect to show in their own and their children's health. The Biologists noted that the increase in health and vitality of the families was surprising and impressive and also the improvement in the relationships observable between children and parents and wives and husbands. It seemed to them that the mothers remained to endure the hard work and the hardships because they were growing fresh healthy food for their own children, and, at the same time, were learning so many new skills and acquiring new interests. Their self-esteem and joy in life was increased by the development of their potential capabilities. Their lives had become fuller and more significant – an increase, apparently, on what membership of the Centre had already affected.

Then came the Battle of Britain. Bromley Common was close to Biggin Hill, the RAF fighter base which the Luftwaffe were trying to put out of action. Dr Williamson decided to call it a day. They began to prepare to leave but, before they could do so, Oakley House was commandeered by the RAF and they were forced to disperse in a hurry. The farm stock was quickly sold. A week later, the farm sheds, dairy, garages, and greenhouses were destroyed by enemy action and a neighbour's cow killed. Many of the Centre records were also destroyed, although Dr Pearse had had time to analyse some of the figures.

7. The Centre school

Shortly before the outbreak of war, families had begun to discuss the possibility of starting a school for the children aged four to seven, (the Infant School age group). Soon after the reopening in 1946, the subject was brought up again and the Biologists were consulted. It was found that the Centre management was willing to pay half the salary of a qualified school teacher to direct the school in the mornings on condition that she acted as a member of the Centre staff in the afternoon, making the 'instruments of health' available to all the children and not only to those on the school roll. It was agreed that the school should use the Centre building rent free during the mornings when it was otherwise unoccupied.

There were several families with a child rising five whom they would shortly be legally bound to send to a school of some sort, and they were impatient to get the Centre school started. At the first meeting of these parents and other interested families, it was agreed that the responsibility for the overall direction of the school should be taken by a committee consisting of both parents of all the children attending the school. This committee should have a secretary and treasurer elected to serve for two years; the meetings should be chaired by the members of the committee in rotation.

At one meeting, the question of fees was discussed. The problem they found difficult to solve was whether dues should be paid per child or per family. Argument continued for an hour or more. Why should a family with only one child pay the same as a family that might be sending three children to the school at one time? No vote was called because the committee was conducted on the Quaker system where decisions are taken only when all present agree. Then a mother with an only child spoke, 'Just as we parents need and are able to make friends in the Centre, so do our children. Mr and Mrs X have six children. It's not so important for their younger ones to have the school because they have each other to learn from. We have only one and he needs friends much more than theirs do. So we are quite ready to pay as much as Mr and Mrs X. And anyway, they have more expenses with their six than we have with our one. Our school is going to be a family school just as the Centre is a family club... It's plain we should have a family subscription just as we have for Centre membership.' There was unanimous agreement. It was decided that each family should pay five shillings and six pence weekly.

At another meeting it was decided that children of three and a half or over attending the Centre nursery whose parents and the nursery supervisor agreed were ready for the next stage should be admitted to the school, and that the children of new member-families aged three and a half or over should be eligible only after a three-months attendance in the nursery.

What kind of school did these families want? Probably many were unable to say in any detail but it seems that they were agreed, as a former member of the school committee has recently recalled, that they wanted a school that 'continued the nurseries'. They had been impressed by how capable, confident and happy their children had become since attending the Centre nurseries. They had watched the children learning through observation of the spontaneous inventions of others and trying out their own ideas whenever the desire and the opportunity coincided. They had seen how assiduously a child will practise a skill it is keen to master and how quickly it learns, when it is free to learn when and how it will. They were perhaps less inclined to worry about their children being left behind in the educational rat race than parents are today, and many of them were aware that all-round physical, mental and emotional development is more important than prowess in the three 'R's. They knew that, if these five year olds went to the state Infant School, it would be around four in the afternoon before they could get to the Centre, and feared that the children, tired after the long day in strange and bewildering – and perhaps frustrating – circumstances, would be unable to make effective use of the facilities for the all-round self-education that were to be found in the Centre building. They wanted their children to be able to continue to learn at their own pace, and for learning to be anxiety-free for as long as possible. Some, knowing how dominant the teacher is in the classroom, feared that dislike or fear of her or fear of failing to come up to her expectations might kill their children's appetite for book-learning.

Eventually just the right teacher for the Centre school was found, a gifted, sensitive and imaginative young woman. She made it possible for each child to work individually, giving them just the right amount of assistance, at the right moment. Elsie Purser noted that 'Elizabeth [Neave] did not talk to the children much, so the children had to come to her.'

The first hour of every morning was spent by the children playing out of doors or on the covered playground with such things as small bicycles, scooters, roller skates, wood, saws, hammers and nails, sand and water and other materials for construction. Then they moved upstairs to one end of the Long Room. They put out the chairs and tables and the trolleys of equipment. This was similar to that used in a modern well-equipped Infant School but included Montessori apparatus. The method of learning reading and writing developed by Marion Cranitch in her Infant School in Goole was used: the children were encouraged to make books of their own; they drew pictures; the teacher added words or phrases as instructed by the child, and, finally, 'stories' were written by the children round the drawings and the child could read what he had written. Each child had a large book of plain paper for this work.

A Bedford station wagon driven by a member who was a retired bus driver was used to collect some of the children who lived in the furthest parts of the 'District' or whose mothers had a small baby, or had to take

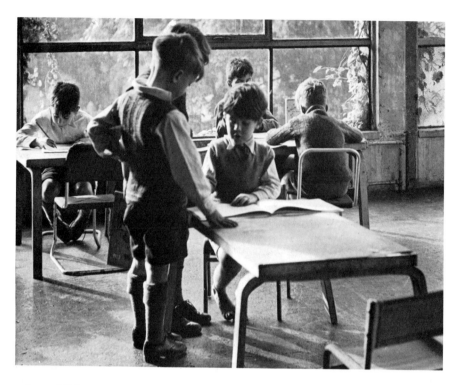

other children to school in the opposite direction. The van also took them home at midday. The children usually returned at 2pm with their mothers. In the afternoons, the children could use the learners' pool under supervision and the gymnasium or they could continue doing what they had been doing in the morning in the Long Room, reading, writing, painting, drawing, modelling, and such like. Often there were mothers available who would read stories or play the piano for 'dancing'. At 4pm, members' children attending other schools would begin to come in, extending the age group upwards, and all through the afternoon, mothers and a few fathers and adolescents would be using the Centre – active in their own way. The school was in the community, not shut away in an artificial world of its own.

The school continued to flourish until the final closure of the Centre, when it contained about 60 pupils. After the closure, some of the parents carried on the school in a Conservative Club hall, but because of the inadequacy of the premises and because they could not afford a trained teacher, it became a school for under-fives, classified later as a Pre-school Playgroup, and only came to an end in 1975. It was a Centre member, Mrs Gibson, who had been employed to look after the equipment and clean the premises when the school was in the Centre, who acted as the Supervisor of the playgroup for the whole 25 years.

8. The evening nursery

A member of the nursery staff watched over babies under two (or still able to sleep comfortably in their prams) from 8pm to 10pm.

9. Nursery teas

Dr Pearse enlisted the assistance, on a rota, of the mothers of the nursery children in preparing an afternoon meal for the children. This preparation took place in the kitchen alongside the cafeteria and therefore in full view of anyone interested. The menus and recipes followed were suggested by Dr Pearse, and use was made, whenever possible, of the organically grown vegetables and fruit from the Centre farm. The Doctor had a special liking for spinach which was not always shared by the children. (In the light of present knowledge, one might almost believe this was an instance of the instinctive wisdom of babies!) For some of the staff, the sight of the wholesale spooning of food into the mouths of the captive children went a little against the grain.

Dr Pearse found the preparation of the nursery teas a practical way of getting information on nutrition and on skilful 'conservative' cooking across to parents who, like most town-dwellers at the time, were ignorant of these things and at the mercy of advertisements and the corner shop-keeper who tended to sell the least perishable types of food.

10. Aids to self-service

The principle of self-service that was followed in all the planning of ways of making the building and its equipment and facilities available to members was not only for the sake of economy; it was part of the attempt to facilitate spontaneity and freedom of choice, awareness and responsibility and to decrease enforced dependence on others. In this country, self-service did not begin to become the common method of getting food and other goods to the customer until well after the 1939–45 war. The Biologists wrote:

> A healthy individual does not like to be waited on – Servants tend to bind and circumscribe action, for their presence makes inevitable the establishment of a routine that only too often rebounds upon their employers.*

So the staff of the Centre was small on principle. The installation of methods of self-service was expensive however; many items of equipment, large and small, had to be especially designed and manufactured since at the time there was nothing suitable on the market. For example '£60 [£1,800 now?] had to be paid for the first mould for an unbreakable plastic plate/saucer; in use it was found to chip readily and had to be

* 1943, p. 75

replaced by a metal one, for the initial pattern of which a further similar sum had to be paid.'

Lucy Crocker's cabinets for storing and displaying the equipment on loan to the children while they were in the building have been mentioned. They were designed to facilitate the exercise of choice and responsibility by the children as well as to reduce the routine work of the Curator of the Instruments of Health and her assistants. They could be locked and wheeled into corners or passages, to make the space available for different uses at other times of the day. It will be recalled that the idea was to make each compartment or pigeon hole fit as closely as possible to the shape of the object it was intended to house. I remember accompanying Lucy to a local pattern-maker to discuss her plans and place the order.

It quickly became a tradition with the children to leave their signed 'tickets' in the pigeon holes and, on returning the objects to their places, to 'post' the tickets into a box provided. Thus, it was made easy for the children to exercise responsibility for the equipment and to play a part in making it continuously available to all – including themselves again on the morrow. Many of the tickets were incompletely filled in and, no doubt, a few never found their way into the boxes after use; it is also likely that occasionally the things were borrowed without the permissive ticket. This would have caused our records of the childrens' doings to be incomplete, but it was no reason for scrapping the system. Its main purposes were achieved. Incidentally I cannot recall having to spend any time at all in collecting up the toys and equipment from around the building and returning them to the cabinets, either during the afternoon or at the end of it.

Talking to a former member recently, I heard that, on paying the fee of two old pence for a hot bath, it was usual to be handed bath-cleaning materials together with the key in order that one could clean the bath after – and also, if one wished, before – using it.

The cafeteria was furnished with a self-service counter but the kitchen was staffed by paid employees. Only when the preparations for a party were under way or when mothers were preparing the nursery teas did members themselves use the kitchen. Washing up was done, as far as it was possible in those days, by machine. The small tray-like plate/saucer, such as is sold today for tele-viewers' snacks, was more useful in the Centre than the largish trays provided in today's self-service restaurants; it was adequate for the food on sale – no complete dinners were provided. These trays were easily washed up and they saved on crockery. Also they took up far less space on the tables which were small and designed to seat the maximum number of people in an informal arrangement.

11. **Parties**

One member, Ron Mulvaney, is reputed to have said, 'The Centre is our front room.' Gladys Coring remembers, 'Some of us who didn't have good facilities in our own homes used to get together to entertain each other in the Centre... I used to bring my brother to the Centre.' Others remember family anniversary parties.

Unfortunately for a time after the war, a rule had to be made limiting visitors to one per member at one time, though I guess that exceptions were made when the gatekeeper, Mr Hayes, knew the proposed visitors sufficiently well. The trouble had been that non-members would hang around at the entrance until they had persuaded a young member to 'sign them in' and then behave in a manner that was unacceptable to the membership.

Two or three enormous parties were organised annually by members. I remember a New Year Party and, for children, a Christmas Party, and a Centre Birthday Party in May or June every year, and in the post-war period, a St Valentine's Dance was organised by younger members. These were all exhilarating and most memorable experiences. 600 members attended the Centre's second Birthday Party, which was held on the Saturday of the week of the Coronation of George VI. These occasions involved many weeks of preparation including the decoration of the building – all part of the fun when done in a group.

The following is a brief description of events at the Centre during 'Coronation Week' from the 1937 Annual Report:

> The Centre's propaganda programme of activities for the Week had involved three months' preparation by its members, and included circularizing the district twice (5,000 families) to invite non-member families to visit the Centre during the week. The entertainments arranged for the visitors included performances by the Dramatic Society and the Concert Party, billiards and badminton matches, diving displays and dancing each night to the Centre Band. During the week about 1,000 people took advantage of our invitation.
>
> On Coronation Day itself, a Children's Fair was held in the grounds and was attended by 350 children of members and 405 children of non-members. The tea was arranged and prepared by a committee of members, and the 750 children served themselves. Over 100 members took part in the construction, erection and running of the Fair apparatus, the carpentry alone involving the leisure time of thirty members for three months.

Apart from this, every Saturday night, the regular dance in the Long Room filled the building with a party atmosphere. As Wally and Olive Arnold put it, 'Saturday was the big night; it wasn't organised, it just came out from nowhere.'

12. Sunday morning swimming (7am – 9am) and occasional Sunday evening activities were organised by members who took responsibility for the building during those hours.

13. A trampoline

This was copied from one he saw used by acrobats in a variety show and built and set up in the playground by Dr Robert Bolton, who from 1935 to 1938 was one of the four physicians on the staff. He went backstage and learned how to construct it from the artistes, and then made one with the enthusiastic help of some of the members. He built a frame in the playground to which it could be attached and set it up whenever he or a deputy could spare the time to supervise its use.

Mrs Ethel Gardiner remembered that the boxers, wrestlers and divers used the trampoline. 'I was a diver', she said, 'and I used it a few times.' The children loved it. Adge Elven said to me recently, 'The first time I realised I had complete control over my body was when doing somersaults on the trampoline. We helped Doc. Bolton to build it and he helped us to use it.'

14. In the playground before the war, there were much used **cricket practice nets.**

15. After the war, there was a **junior cycling group** and a very enthusiastic **football club**. Both these used the gymnasium for exercise and training.

16. Children's music-making

I remember very well Mr Hirschfelt's music-maker. He was a refugee from National Socialism in Germany, and had been a member of the Bauhaus, the headquarters of a group of original and creative artists and craftsmen collected around himself by the architect Walter Gropius in the days of the Weimar Republic. He had invented a way of enabling children who had had no musical instruction of any kind to make music together. During 1939, he often came to the Centre in the afternoon and would sit down in the Long Room and play his concertina, having set out beside him an assortment of his home-made wind and percussion instruments, such as bamboo pipes and wooden xylophones. In front of him he had an apparatus, the 'music maker', consisting of poles which he could lever up in turn by means of pedals; the tops of the poles were painted in various colours which corresponded to colours painted on the keys or around the stops of the instruments. Children observing the rules of the game could make music with him, making sounds that harmonised with the melody he was playing.

17. From time to time a **discussion group** flourished, using one of the committee rooms.

18. Throughout most of 1948, a **monthly magazine** called the *Guinea Pig* was produced by and for members. It was the brain child of 'Nobby' Clarke, a young plumber. Early in 1949, it was succeeded by *The Centre* which continued until the Centre closed in March 1950, under the editorship of Ron Goldsmith, a hairdresser with his own business. A variety of talent was forthcoming for these enterprises, – artists, typists, photographers and reporters, and anyone could, of course, contribute, including children.

19. **Dr Anni Noll** was Dr Pearse's trusted and loved assistant during the whole of the four years up to the outbreak of war. There was more than enough work for two women doctors and she was a brilliant paediatrician. Unfortunately for the Centre, she married during the war, and, since she preferred to spend her evenings with her husband, was no longer available to work at the Centre. Olive Smith who was 15 in 1939 has told me that she was so impressed with the sex-education talk Dr Noll gave her that she remembered it almost word for word and has frequently used it herself on occasions when sex education was called for.

20. **Dressmaking classes**

These were conducted by Margaret Collins, a member of long standing, who had been a dressmaker, had trained as a nurse during the war and, after the Centre reopened, was in charge of the babies' and toddlers' nursery. The management invested in three or four sewing machines and a couple of cutting-out tables, designed as usual to fold up out of the way when not in use. When Mrs Collins was unavailable, members helped each other with advice.

Throughout the life of the Centre, members shared their skills with each other on a casual and informal basis.

A clothing exchange was organised by members during the post-war period.

21. **A 25-minute film**, *The Centre*, was commissioned by the Foreign Office for showing abroad. It was directed by Paul Rotha. Centre members provided the cast. The first public showing was in July 1949 at the Odeon in Peckham. H M Queen Mary and Clement Atlee, the Prime Minister, were in the audience and visited the Centre afterwards. It was Queen Mary's second visit; the first was in 1939 when she gave a generous donation. (On that occasion I was with the splashing children in the babies' pool when she was conducted along the narrow passage beside the pool. She stopped and watched and did not seem to share my

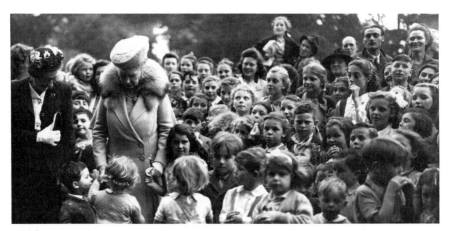

Queen Mary's second visit

fear that her beautiful velvet coat would be spoilt by the water.) The film was shown all over the world and in eight different languages, in two cinemas in Paris, also in Cardiff, Cambridge and, for six days, in Coventry.

22. The Post-war resurrection

The following account of how this came about was written for the *Bulletin of the PHC* of May 1949:

> The Centre closed in 1939 when war broke out. It re-opened largely through the remarkable persistence of 500 of its member families – in 1945. War changed the Family Health Club into a factory that made spare parts for bombers. The Centre's records were burnt when part of the Bromley Home Farm was gutted. Nearly a quarter of the Peckham houses were demolished. Some of the Centre members were killed. Yet war – with seven years of disintegration – failed to destroy the continuity of the Peckham Experiment.
>
> During the war, news began to filter through from some of the member-families, and, as time went on, there was increasing evidence that, to some of the families at any rate, peace was beginning to mean, not only family reunion and the rebuilding of a home, but a return to what can perhaps loosely be described as the 'Peckham way of life'. How strong would that urge prove to be? How many families would feel this way when war was over? These were questions which the doctors, concerned to know how deeply the 'Peckham' idea had rooted itself, frequently asked themselves.
>
> In the end, it was old Mr Hayes, the gatekeeper, who touched off the 'Get the Centre back' movement. He'd joined the Centre in '35, the year it opened, and was proud of proving that his membership number was only 39. The people called him 'Baldie', and everyone knew him. When the factory took over, he was kept on as gatekeeper. In off-duty hours

he often met old Centre friends, and he took care to keep the news circulating.

The Centre's list of addresses had gone up in flames; it would have been out of date anyway, for most of the people had moved. One day Mr Hayes bought himself a penny notebook, and set himself the hard task of making a new list. The idea caught on and spread. Quite soon a meeting place was needed, and so Elsie Purser, another Centre member, offered her home as headquarters. It was the urge to get the Centre started again – to live the fuller life they were all missing so badly – which brought her back to her war–damaged house in Peckham from a nicer home in Streatham. The Centre was held by the Government, but the hope of getting it released was so deeply felt, and so commonly shared, by those who had experienced Centre life that it drew many families away from pleasanter districts, back to live in Peckham.

Mrs Purser's sitting room soon became too small. The hat went round, a church hall was hired, and a meeting held which 100 people attended. By this time, the families were in touch with Amy Moor, the Centre receptionist, and Donald Wilson, the manager. By the summer of 1945, the list of family names was 500 strong. The people felt the time had come to get help from the doctors. Again they hired a hall, and they sent a formal invitation to Dr Pearse and Dr Scott Williamson to come and talk to them. Fifteen hundred men, women and children attended this meeting. It took the doctors nearly eight hours to meet them all and hear all their stories. Dr Williamson gave them the answer they all sought 'You are a community,' he said. 'Demand the place back. You'll get it!'

Before the meeting was over, a petition, intended for presentation to the Prime Minister, was drafted. Six hundred copies were printed and signed, and one was waiting in the locker of every Member of Parliament on the day of the re-opening of the House. That was how a nucleus of the pre-war membership (about 75 per cent) regained the Family Health Club. The Centre building was in a sorry mess. Oil and grease had been ground into the cork floors. Heavy benches and a flood had damaged the gymnasium floor. The great glass windows were dirty, cracked or broken. It looked shabby and desolate, but nobody cared. *They had the Centre back again!*

Within eleven days, the Centre gave its famous self-organised and never-to-be-forgotten party. All the families came, and invitations were sent to the Centre's many friends.

There was still no glass round the swimming pool, but the concrete with which it had been filled, in order to hold the factory benches, had been hacked out. The water was in again, deeply green and inviting. Children struggled into bathing suits, and as the first boy took the high dive, the people who thronged round the pool laughed as they drew back from the splash. Centre life had re-started. And members were celebrating not an end, but a beginning of their future together.

Visitors speak every language and are of every colour, but a question they often ask is, 'Just why did you want your Centre back so badly?' When a newspaper man put it to Olive Fee (now Olive Smith), one night – her husband John had refused a better job, and a nicer house in another

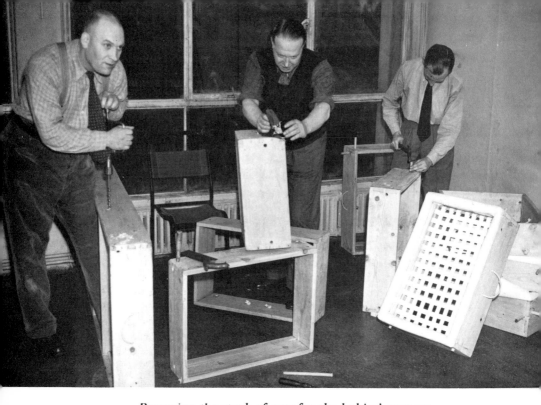

Renewing the stock of cots for the babies' nursery

Many offered their time and skills to clean, repair and refurbish the building

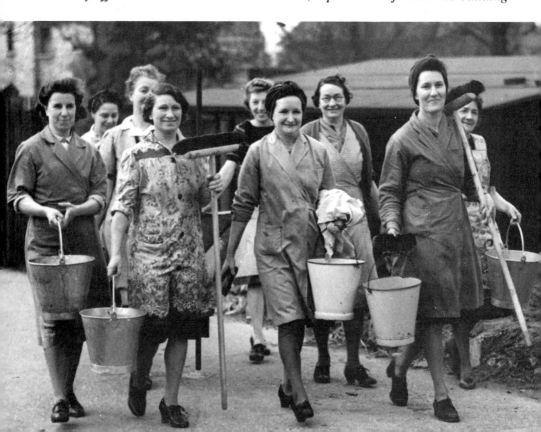

suburb – she replied for the whole family. 'Well, you see, we're all here together. There's something for all of us.'

Members answer the visitor's questions according to their age, their temperament, and the way they happen to live. It is only when you add all the answers that you begin to glimpse the whole picture, and then it becomes clear to you that when families get together, in an environment that is rich in opportunity for all of them, a force of incalculable power is released. They begin to live. They begin to adventure. Physique improves, and the mind starts to explore. Initiative develops, and the material difficulties, still sadly evident in the lives of the 'Peckham' member-families, no longer control the situation.

Not all the families experience this enrichment. If the capacity to 'grow' through opportunity has died within them, the Centre cannot bring it to life again, and for those no longer capable of development, 'Peckham' has little to offer. Happily they are in the minority. Amongst the majority, there is evidence that family health and happiness are cultivatable, and it is evidence so strong, and so significant, that it holds out great hope for all families everywhere. It is for the sake of all the nation's families – and not just for the fortunate few at 'Peckham' – that the 'Peckham' research goes on.

Dr J Greenwood Wilson, Cardiff's Medical Officer of Health wrote:

To attend the big party at this huge glass building of so unusual design, held to commemorate its release from war-time requisitioning, was an unforgettable experience. The radiance in the faces of the people seemed something more than the jollity of the party spirit.

Chapter 5

Findings

The findings regarding the physical condition of the 500 families examined during the first eighteen months of the main experiment are reported in *Biologists in Search of Material* (1938), and of the total of 1,206 families examined in the four and a half pre-war years, in *The Peckham Experiment* (1943).

Scott Williamson and Innes Pearse were looking for health and hoping to find it. Few if any of the people examined had joined the Centre in order to obtain advice or treatment or because they wanted a medical check up. (I imagine the latter phrase was never heard in those days, at least in Peckham.) They had joined for the keep-fit or games facilities, the play opportunities for children, or the nurseries for babies. Very few considered themselves to be anything worse than temporarily a bit under the weather and they were all going about their daily tasks and carrying on with their jobs. Yet the results of the laboratory tests and the thorough examination by a doctor revealed the surprising fact that out of a total of 3,911 individuals of all ages examined, only 358 (less than ten per cent) had nothing the matter with them. All the rest had some physiological defect or deficiency – some objectively ascertainable disorder, and many had more than one. The conditions listed in *Biologists in Search of Material* ranged from the most trivial to the most serious, from corns, deformed toes, decayed teeth, and varicose veins to heart and kidney disorders, seriously high blood pressure and cancer.[*]

Public reaction, when these figures were published, was one of astonishment even incredulity, but, since then, similar figures have been obtained when a number of people presumed to have been healthy have been examined.[†]

The Peckham figures were further analysed according to whether or not the individual *felt* unwell. Of all the individuals over the age of five discovered to have a clinically recognisable disorder of some sort, only 65 per cent were aware of having anything wrong. The rest maintained that they were 'quite well'. They regarded such trials as catarrh, bunions, constipation or lassitude as normal and to be expected. Some had really serious disorders and were quite ignorant of it. As the Biologists wrote, these figures provide evidence of the fact that many serious maladies go through an initial stage in which the sufferer is unlikely to realise that anything is wrong with him, and also that there are many debilitating

[*] A concise account of the medical condition of the member-families as revealed by the overhaul is to be found in Barlow (1988) pp. 83–86
[†] In 1961 in the USA and in 1970 in Southwark, England

physiological disorders from which people may suffer for years without being aware of it. One wonders how it can be that a person can remain for so long unaware that he is ill. The answer lies, they say, in the wonderful ability of the body as a whole to keep going in spite of having faulty parts. The body has reserves of materials and energy which are, in health, available to it for use in an emergency or when a challenge is encountered, but, when it is occupied in compensating for some disorder or deficiency, these reserves are being used up in order to keep the body chugging along and on an even keel; therefore they are no longer available on occasions when increased effort or activity is necessary or desired. The Biologists write that the body's power of compensation is valuable in that it allows an injured part time to recover, but, if it is used other than temporarily, it can be dangerous because 'it masks the injury and wear and tear and postpones the moment when the necessity for doing something about it becomes apparent.'*

At the 'family consultation', the information obtained through the overhaul was given to the husband and wife together. This, Williamson and Pearse thought, may have been a cause of the frequency with which the doctors' advice was sought regarding treatment: one or other partner would usually enquire what could be done to remedy any troubles revealed by the overhaul. In the case of serious disorder, Innes Pearse and Scott Williamson, both of whom had held posts in various London hospitals, often knew where the most precise diagnosis and effective treatment could be obtained, and would send the member with a letter to a particular specialist or hospital. They would advise people with minor maladies where to seek treatment or to consult their general practitioner or 'panel' doctor.

It was found advisable to offer a health overhaul to all members on discharge from hospital, for after a period of sickness and inactivity, they were sometimes found to be in a low state caused by disorders and deficiencies that they had not had at their previous overhaul. By this means, the Centre doctors were able to check up on the results of the treatment for which the member had entered hospital. If it had not been effective, they did their best to see that successful treatment was obtained.

I remember very clearly a small example of the Biologists' faith in the body's power to heal itself. A six year old boy spent some time in hospital. When he came out, his feet were almost completely flat. I have a mental picture of him with his flat feet in the gym. He loved playing in the gym, and, as the days passed, I remember that the arches of his feet rose up until they were perfectly formed. No wedges on his shoes, or foot supports (which are likely, in my experience, to permanently weaken or deform the feet) – simply barefoot play in a place where there was opportunity for climbing, jumping, running, for as long or as little as he wanted.

* 1943

The Biologists found that there was no provision by the medical services for the treatment of many minor ailments and also incipient diseases such as, for example, the early stages of high blood pressure, kidney disorder and anaemia. The reason was no doubt partly because people suffering from such defects rarely sought treatment so that neither general practitioners nor hospital staff encountered many cases and as a result saw no need to make provision for them. Whatever the reason, Drs Williamson and Pearse found it necessary to give a certain amount of treatment in spite of their original intention not to do so.

Anaemia in varying degrees was a common condition disclosed by the laboratory tests. Out of 1,660 individuals examined during the first eighteen months, 657 had low haemoglobin values. Some were very low by any standard and, with regard to the rest, Scott Williamson and Innes Pearse were unwilling to accept as normal the figure generally accepted by the medical profession (which was, incidentally, based on tests made on hospital patients), since they found that most people were capable of reaching and maintaining a considerably higher level than this 'normal' figure, after having been treated with iron (often combined with liver extract or vitamins and occasionally, in particularly stubborn cases, with liver injections) and when they had been cured of accompanying dis-orders and had begun to lead a more physically, mentally or socially active life. The figures showed that low haemoglobin was much more frequent in women of childbearing age than in older women or men. Substances such as iron and vitamins were supplied free to pregnant women and charged to 'research'. At that time. knowledge of the body's needs with regard to vitamins and minerals had not progressed far. The Peckham Biologists' actions, based on such knowledge as was available, plus their own insight, proved to have most beneficial results. Members were amazed at how well and active women could be during their pregnancies, for the general expectation was to feel tired and even ill.*

Infestation by thread worms was found to be common in children and sometimes appeared to be the cause of anaemia and general malnutrition. Ethelyn Hazell recalls that one or two of the children who went to live at Oakley House on the outbreak of war were badly afflicted with worms.

> One in particular was absolutely riddled with them: she wet the bed, slept badly, had a lot of crying fits and dreams at night, and was generally 'naughty' and difficult. She needed to pass water frequently and there used to be a rush if anyone saw the child running almost with her legs crossed trying not to wet her pants. She was treated for worms and I saw the potty in which she passed her stool after the treatment and the sight was quite incredible. After that and following her follow-up treatment, she was a completely different child and became fit and happy.

The Biologists learned to recognise seriously affected children from their appearance and their behaviour (nervousness, inability to concentrate

---

* See members' testimonies in Chapter 8

and to play with enjoyment). They would ask the parents to bring specimens of their child's stools to the laboratory for investigation. They devised an effective and reliable treatment and if possible the whole family was treated. Allan Pepper, for many years Hon. Secretary and then Chairman of the executive committee of the Pioneer Health Centre Ltd. and who, as a young man, spent as much time as he could spare listening to Scott Williamson and Innes Pearse, recalls:

> Dod (as Scott Williamson was known to his friends), Dod told me that one day Lucy Crocker said to him, 'Young Jimmy there has got rid of his worms, hasn't he?' 'Yes, how did you know?' 'His behaviour – his action pattern – has changed.' And she gave details.

In the annual report for 1937, Williamson and Pearse wrote:

> Our experience from the second family overhauls of some 230 families indicates that the majority of minor maladies that can be cured remain cured, and that a great number of major maladies that can be alleviated remain alleviated.

This had not been the case during the three years of the pilot scheme (1926–9). They doubted whether periodic medical examination designed to disclose disorders and to remedy them by clinical means would, by itself, lead to a decrease in sickness or an increase in health, but:

> ... experience has shown that enhanced vitality and a wider measure of freedom from sickness can be attained through periodic health overhaul of families *in the circumstances provided by the Centre.*[*]

It was obvious to the Biologists that people need to be as free as possible of physical disorders and deficiencies if they are to take advantage of the opportunity to develop health in themselves. Therefore, for the sake of the research as well as for the sake of the individuals concerned, they found themselves forced to spend a great deal of time and thought and energy on helping people to free themselves of impediments to health.

It is interesting to note that both before and after the war, an osteopath spent an evening a week working in the Centre. Pre-war it was a Dr Oswald Dieter. It was he who gave the Biologists an interesting bit of information. He said that about 24 hours before labour begins, all a woman's ligaments loosen. Gladys Coring tells that, on one occasion, she was most impressed by Dr Williamson's prophetic powers when, the day before her daughter was born, he came up to her in the cafeteria, put his arm round her shoulders and then said, 'We'll not see *you* in the pool tomorrow.' Later, when Mary Langman was running the dairy farm at Oakley House, her herdsman told her that you could always tell when calving is imminent by feeling the cow's ligaments.

* * * * *

* 1943, p. 116

Unfortunately the stir caused by the publication of their findings concerning the state of ill-health of the population of Peckham caused some people to jump to the conclusion that their aim in setting up the experiment was to show the value of early diagnosis and preventative medicine. In truth, these discoveries were quite incidental to their main purpose which was to undertake an investigation into the nature of positive health and into the nature of the circumstances in which health can be cultivated by the inhabitants of cities and conurbations.

Scott Williamson and Innes Pearse became aware of a fact that, to this day, frequently escapes people; it is that the absence of disease and disorder is not the same thing as health. The two are utterly different. People have wondered why they did not try to prove the Centre's value by comparing the number of people without ascertainable disorder at the first and second overhauls. Had they done so, the figures obtained would have done no more than demonstrate the increase in the number of members without a recognisable physical disorder or deficiency. They would have given no idea of the increase in the physical, mental and emotional vitality of individuals or of the quality of their behaviour and their relationships with each other and with their environment as a whole. Health cannot be measured. It is revealed, for example, not so much by the *amount* of social, physical or mental activity undertaken by a person as by its *quality*. It was found that the ten per cent of members who were, at the time of their first overhaul, free of recognisable disorders, were not necessarily outstanding examples of vitality or good physical or social judgement; the Biologists did not classify this ten per cent as healthy. As we have seen, they never labelled individual people healthy or unhealthy. Health, they said, is not a state; it is a process. A person may manifest health at some times and in some situations and not in others, for health is manifested in a person's relationship with his social and physical environment, and the nature of this relationship depends partly on the past and present nature of his environment.

By the time I had got to know the Centre well, when it had been open for a year and a half, and many members had been wholly or partially relieved of the deficiencies or disorders from which they had been suffering when they joined, the picture was beginning to be one of health. I say this because I remember many people, particularly children but whole families too, who seemed to me to behave in general in a way that could be described as healthy in the 'Peckham' sense. They seemed to me to act appropriately to the needs of the total situation in which they found themselves at any moment, instead of reacting to one or other of its elements only. They seemed to be aware of their own needs as whole personalities and also of the needs of the greater wholes of which they were parts – family, group of friends or play companions, and the society of the Centre as a whole. It seemed to me that they acted both with spontaneity and with discrimination, and to be well on their way to acquiring good judgement in many and varied fields of activity – in the only possible way, which is the exercise of their faculty for judgement. As I described in Chapter 3 and describe again in Chapter 9, the behaviour of the children in the gym and the swimming pool was a very easily recognisable example of healthy behaviour – within a limited sphere of activity. Their movements were precise and effective and economical of effort, yet smooth and graceful; and not only did each individual demonstrate superb physical co-ordination and judgement, but he was also acting as part of an integrated and harmonious whole.

Here are a few figures relating to the use of the Centre. They were printed in the Annual Report for 1937 (not published until 1938). The number of members coming into the Centre during one week in April 1938 was recorded:

Monday	591
Tuesday	650
Wednesday	759
Thursday	801
Friday	865
Saturday	960
Total for the week	4,626
Average	771

On Wednesday, the total of 759 individuals was made up of:

Women	329
Babies (under 5)	41
Men	231
Children (5–16)	158

The number of paid-up member-families on the books at the time was 600.

The facilities used by members during a single day at the Centre were also roughly recorded as follows:

	Adults	Children
Cafeteria	280	54
Swimming (Large pool)	73	46
Swimming (Small pool)	—	13
Table Tennis	22	11
Darts	24	11
Billiards	42	22
Badminton	20	16
Gymnasium	25	42
Long Room (Social & dancing)	140	90

Whist.	36	–
Crafts.	–	13
Dance	112	–
Band Rehearsal	9	–
Nursery	–	26
Night Nursery	–	3

	Adults	Children
Medical Dept. appointments . .	63	20
Medical casual consultations . .	42	22

It was recorded that 157 married women learned to swim during the first four years that the Centre was open. As the staff observed and as the former members I have contacted recently remember with pleasure, they made acquaintances and life-long friends through swimming, or playing badminton, and enjoyed the opportunity to sit together afterwards in the cafeteria over a cup of tea while – their babies and toddlers safe and happy in the nurseries – they awaited the arrival of older children from school. These relationships often led to friendships between whole families: holidays were spent together and the children grew up together. These family friendships are recalled with gratitude. Some have survived to this day. A family that emigrated to Canada when the Centre closed in 1951 returned twenty years later on a visit and told Dr Pearse that they had made the journey mainly in order to see their old Centre friends again.

The following story was related to Allan Pepper by Scott Williamson. One day, he met a member on the stairs at the Centre, stopped and asked her how she was doing. 'I am so happy,' was the reply, 'I have so may friends.' 'But surely you had friends before you joined the Centre.' 'No, not real friends, not like these. I never made friends before.' The staff were amazed to discover how lonely people in Peckham were. Former members I have recently contacted have volunteered the fact that membership of the Centre gave them friends for the first time in their adult lives. Continuity of acquaintanceship between families must have had its effect combined with the opportunity to work together on initiatives such as the formation of new clubs, the production of dramatic entertainments, the organisation of and preparation for parties or weekend camping.

Some newly joined young couples suffered from shyness and lack of confidence to such an extent that it was found by the Biologists to be a mistake to introduce them to a well-established member-family sitting near them in the cafeteria, however lonely and out of things they might appear to be feeling. It seemed merely to drive home to them the fact of their social inadequacy and to increase their misery. It proved to be better to wait, hoping that some activity might prove to be irresistible or an acquaintanceship spring up spontaneously. One former member recalled that at first she and her husband 'did not find people were friendly, and we left'. Some months later they rejoined, began to play badminton and made friends with whom they have kept in touch ever since.*

The Borough of Camberwell, of which Peckham was a part, contained swimming pools, playing fields and opportunities for social and cultural activities, but it was discovered that surprisingly few of the members were using these facilities when they joined.

The first 200 or so families to join were slow to make use of the pool, the gym and the badminton court; they sat over tea or beer at the tables around the pool or played whist. The Biologists wondered if the sight of skilled swimmers, divers or gymnasts enjoying the amenities would be encouraging. So they invited some enthusiasts to visit the Centre and use the well-equipped pool and gymnasium; but it did not have the desired effect. It worked only for the few who had some confidence in their own proficiency. For the large majority, it appeared to have an inhibiting effect. The spectacle of expertise did not stimulate them to try to imitate it; it only made them more conscious of their own lack of skill. It was enjoyable to watch and that was all. So invitations to the experts were discontinued.

Attempts at moral persuasion also failed. It appeared that people distrusted and resisted the least display of paternalism. Scott Williamson suspected this to be a sign of health. So the only course open to him was to sit back and wait. Gradually brave spirits who could hardly swim or not at all joined the more skilled in the pool, in full view, as it was, of everybody. People found, as Gladys Coring recalls†, that they soon forgot the spectators. The glass wall provided a sufficient barrier (perhaps because it excluded the chance of hearing anyone's comments). The sight of people of all shapes, sizes and ages enjoying the water encouraged the timid and self-conscious, who began to think, 'If she can, why not I?' The same thing happened elsewhere in the building. Gradually people became doers as well as spectators. Members with skills and enthusiasms began to share them with others. If one wanted help, instruction or advice, it was likely that someone would know someone else who could provide it.

Originally it was planned to have a library on the top floor, and a beginning was made with one, but there was little demand. There was a good public library in the Borough, (although at some distance) and to have provided readers with the amount of choice consistent with 'Peckham' principles was out of the question.

* * * * *

At the beginning, a fear was expressed by some of the Centre's well-wishers that the increase in social life would be the cause of broken marriages. It turned out to be quite unfounded. The staff knew of none

* See Chapter 7
† See Chapter 7

during the four pre-war years. After the war there were three divorces, two of which followed on long wartime separation.

On the other hand, the Biologists found plenty of evidence of the restorative effect of Centre life on the marriages of people who, when they joined, had been suffering very unhappy relationships. An example is given in *The Peckham Experiment* (p. 264) of a couple, married for 16 years, who found at last, in the community life of the Centre, scope for their talents and energy. Until they joined, the lack of this had caused them frustration, and unhappiness for themselves and their children.

There was confirmation of Scott Williamson's proposition that 'health ensues when the family is not turned in on itself, but is, instead, exercising its adaptive function on the environment.' When a family keeps itself to itself or has only superficial social relationships, its members tend to be starved of mental and emotional nourishment. When young couples depend entirely on each other for such nourishment, they may find marriage to be a stunting and sterile relationship.

An all-age community evolved. The Centre became an extension of the family's *home* in the sense of a place in which one feels at home, a place with which one is thoroughly familiar and in which one is able to act both spontaneously and effectively. It was like home also in the sense of something one is playing a part in creating. Everybody, young or old, was able to be himself, and this caused a diversity in the Centre life that made it easy to find companions and occupations to one's liking. In time it became a place that the shy and retiring could also enjoy. One former member told me that as a very shy youth who also longed for human warmth, he was happy at the Centre because it was a place 'where you could be alone'. I can understand his feeling. You could sit and watch or wander around on your own without feeling conspicuously solitary and you could enjoy a feeling of being enveloped in a warmly sociable atmosphere without feeling obliged to *be* sociable.

There were members who did not share this community life. Some did not come in often enough to make long-term acquaintances; there were families who belonged only for the sake of the children, the parents visiting it only on the occasion of their medical examination.

But it can be stated with confidence that in very many of the members, a feeling of belonging to a community grew. Gladys Coring insists that a warmer word than 'community' is needed to describe the relationship between the member-families. A contributor to the Bulletin of the Pioneer Health Centre (1949) suggested 'communion'. Elsie Purser, the writer of Chapter 8 who, because of the breadth of her interests and her sociability, had a very large acquaintance among the members, told me,

> It was like belonging to a huge family. We felt responsible for each other. Towards the end, we began to love all the children and not only our own.

When, in 1946, the member-families returned en masse after a gap of seven years, and all the children under ten had either never known the Centre or were not old enough to remember it, it was feared that the chaos of the very first months would be repeated. This did not happen. The children's behaviour was just as acceptable to the adults as it had been during the last three years pre-war. They behaved with quite outstanding responsibility and orderliness. From the time in 1936 when a way had been found of enabling them to use the facilities, like the adults, individually and in their own time, there was virtually no vandalism or rowdy behaviour. It was, in my opinion, due to the children quite as much as to the adults that the all-age community life flourished and that the Centre became and remained a family club in reality.

It has to be admitted that a sense of responsibility for the Centre was not absolutely universal. There were a few families who bilked the Centre of their membership subscriptions for a time. A former member maintains that, at parties or on Saturday nights in the post-war period, a few people took advantage of the minimum staffing and practice of self-service to avoid paying for what they had from the cafeteria.

* * * * *

A reader of my manuscript commented that there was little mention in it of the adolescent age-group. This may have been because I was not aware of them as a separate group. Their behaviour was – like that of most of the pre-adolescents – spontaneous and responsible; they helped themselves to what they needed from the Centre and were content, and they fitted their activities into the whole composed of people of all ages. Like the adults and the children, they acted as individuals, not as a herd, nor did they think of themselves as a group with special requirements. They certainly did not range themselves up against the older generation. Up to the age of 14 or 15 they merged in with the children, and then, imperceptibly, became young adults and acted as such. This was something I had taken for granted; I am glad that my attention has been called to it, for it was, in fact, a most remarkable and interesting phenomenon.

In the post-war period, the conscription of the young men of 18 to 20 upset the balance of ages and sexes in the Centre. A writer in the Bulletin commented:

> In the Centre we see how much is contributed to so many activities by our few young bachelors over the call-up age. As they are not yet involved in family responsibilities, the time and energy they have to give to their chosen activities is invaluable to the general social life. All the more this makes us realise the gap left by the absence of the age-group just below them. The whole of society, younger and older, suffer from the lack of exuberant vitality which is a characteristic condition of that youthful age.

Some parents felt strongly that the two years in the army had a deleterious effect on the young men's development and their future lives. From 15 or 16 onwards they began to feel unsettled, it was said; then when the conscript returned, he tended to get married quickly, often to someone he hardly knew and sometimes unwisely, and to take the first available reasonably well-paid job, however little he was interested in or enjoyed the work.

* * * * *

Now follows an account of some of the Biologists' findings that requires an introduction.

The extant – that is, currently successful – species of animals, birds, fishes and insects possess a kind of wisdom. It is not the kind that is acquired through an individual's experience; it is an inherited wisdom. One could call it biological wisdom. Students of animal behaviour such as Konrad Lorenz have observed and described the manifold ways in which most species act in their own best interests most of the time, because they have built-in instinctive behaviour mechanisms that automatically come into play at appropriate moments and ensure that they will do so.

Wolves provide an example of this biological wisdom. In Canada, a pair of wolves were captured and placed on an island.* The Island was inhabited by a large number of moose. After two or three years the wolves had increased to a small pack. The moose were slightly fewer in number but healthier, as the weaker ones had been weeded out. The leading pair of wolves were the only members of the pack that bred; the others did not mate and helped to feed and care for the young of the leading pair. Behaviour similar to this which promotes quality in the species through restricting quantity has been observed in the wild dog of Africa and in the European fox.

Humans are neither protected nor bound by automatically operating instincts such as these; they are free to act wisely or foolishly, destructively or creatively. But they do possess some basic biological wisdom in the form of instinctive tendencies. One could say, for instance, that it is a wise baby that quickly learns how to suck from the breast efficiently or that takes every opportunity to learn how to balance on his feet and to walk at the moment when the ratio of his strength to his weight, and the distance from the ground of his centre of gravity are most favourable to the learning of these arts.

Our bigger brains do not necessarily help us to act wisely. To be wise we need to integrate our reasoning powers, our instinctive tendencies and our feeling for what is right. Easier said than done. And the circumstances in which we are forced to live are not often conducive to success. Niko Tinbergen has written to the effect that we must try to

* Mech, 1966

make the planners – and other powers that be – understand that, if they are to improve the conditions in which we live,

> ... a better knowledge of the interplay of reason and our deep-rooted, typically human motivations will be essential – knowledge in other words of our true nature.*

Sad to say, very few people agree. Present day scientists, philosophers and people in general all talk as if we were gods, able to make ourselves and our children into whatever we like, and able to adapt to whatever kind of environment we have chanced to manufacture for ourselves. They do not admit to possessing a characteristic human nature. This is so obviously the case that Mary Midgley, senior lecturer in philosophy at the University of Newcastle-upon-Tyne, has felt it necessary to write a book† devoted to the presentation of the case for the *existence* of human nature, and the need to learn about it. She points out that confusion arises over the word instinct. Our basic human instincts are not at all the same thing as the battery of precisely orientated and automatically triggered off instincts possessed by birds and fishes for example. She makes a distinction between 'closed' and 'open' instincts.

> Closed instincts are behaviour patterns fixed genetically in every detail, like the bees' honey dance, some birdsong and the nest-building pattern of weaver birds. Here the same complicated pattern, correct in every detail, will be produced by creatures that have been carefully reared in isolation from any member of their own species and from any helpful conditioning. Such genetic programming takes the place of intelligence; learning is just maturation.

Besides closed instincts, she writes,

> ... an animal's instinctive behaviour includes a number of strong general tendencies to certain *kinds* of behaviour, such as hunting, tree-climbing, washing, singing, or caring for the young... The more complex, the more intelligent, creatures become, the more they are programmed in this general way, rather than in full detail...
>
> With closed instincts, desire and technique go together. A bee cannot just want to dance-in-general; it must dance (and therefore want) only the exact figure that will tell the other bees where it has been. But, as you go up the evolutionary scale, much wider possibilities open. The more adaptable a creature is, the more directions it can go in. So it has more, not less, need for definite tastes to guide it. *What replaces closed instincts, therefore, is not just cleverness, but strong, innate, general desires and interests.* It would be useless to replace the hidebound hunting habits of the wasp simply with the greater intelligence of cats and otters. There must also be a strong general wish to hunt... More obviously still, mammals could not improve on the automatic brood-tending of bees merely by being more intelligent about what benefits infants. They have to *want* to benefit them. And they must want it more, not less, than bees, because

* 1976
† 1977

they are so much freer, and could easily desert their infants if they had a mind to, which is the sort of thing that could simply never occur to a bee. Just in proportion as automatic skills drop off at the higher levels of evolution, innately determined general desires become more necessary. This transition has always been obscured because the word 'instinct' was used for both.*

Open instincts are 'evolutionary devices' without which 'we should grind to a halt', for intelligence by itself cannot replace instinct. 'Instinct covers not just knowing how to do things, but knowing what to do. It concerns ends as well as means.'†

Innate desires and tendencies must have been as essential to the success of early man as they are to the higher animals, but many of those without which our ancestors would not have survived are not needed by civilised man in order to stay alive and procreate. In modern times we have tended to disregard or stifle more and more of them in ourselves and our children. They may seem to us unnecessary and uncalled for in the kind of lives we lead. Scott Williamson held that instincts, in this sense, are a part of the biological wisdom that we could still call on to our advantage, and that, if we wish to flourish as a species, we need to resuscitate the more important of them and allow them to grow strong. He sought to provide the conditions in which they would come to life again.

From my limited knowledge of natural history, it seems to me that, in general, the young of a species spend their time doing what causes them to grow into mature and capable members of their species, and the adults are mainly occupied in furthering the welfare of their offspring and thus ensuring the future of the species. Garden birds provide very obvious examples of devotion to the rearing of the next generation.

To the Peckham Biologists, these two expressions of biological wisdom – activity leading to the full development of one's faculties, and activity promoting the nurture of the next generation – are important manifestations of health in humans. To them, one of the most interesting results of the experiment was that health in this form was manifested after a time by most of the member-families of the Pioneer Health Centre.

Much of this book is devoted to the description of instances of the operation of the first of these two instinctive tendencies. As to the second, I was closer to the children than I was to their parents, but one thing was clear to me; it was that parents who made good use of the Centre enjoyed being parents. By all accounts, they found parenthood satisfying and rewarding. Therefore, if the desire to nurture their children to the best of their ability is instinctive in humans, Centre members would have been likely to demonstrate the fact. And this is what did in effect happen.

* 1977
† *ibid.*

But membership of the Centre not only fanned the desire of parents to nurture their children, it also made it easy for them to do so. In the environment of the Centre, they found it possible to exercise what the Peckham Biologists called 'the faculty for nurture'. The Biologists used the word 'nurture' (rather than bring up, rear, raise, care for or educate) because it denotes precisely the kind of activity that is necessary in order to foster the growth of a body or a personality. Expressed in cold and concise terms, 'nurtural activity' consists in the provision of suitable conditions for growth (nourishing conditions). They used the word 'faculty' in the sense of an innately potential power, natural to humans, but requiring suitable circumstances if it is to develop.

I believe that the condition most essential for the exercise of the faculty for nurture is a faith in the inborn desire of young creatures to grow – to develop their essential human faculties and individual uniqueness and creativity; and that the second most important condition is faith in children's ability to know what to do to that end, as long as they have, from the beginning, consistently suitable opportunities for action.

It is difficult for a family to exercise the faculty for nurture effectively if it is alone in this faith. Ideally it should be shared by the whole of society.

There were, I believe, several reasons why Centre parents acquired the ability to nurture their children well. In the first place, the Peckham Biologists possessed the faith described above and were ready to learn from the children what are 'suitable opportunities for action'. And the pleasure they took in watching children spontaneously exercising and developing their faculties communicated itself to the parents. Through conversations with the Biologists and through watching the activity of other children in the Centre besides their own, Centre parents obtained greater insight into the needs of babies and young children. They came to trust their child's power to grow – like a flower or a tree – and to enjoy watching this happen.

The way in which a Centre mother might be encouraged, right from the beginning, to learn *from the baby* what his needs are is illustrated by Dr Pearse's emphasis on the need to watch the baby's faeces for information as to how well he is digesting his food and when it is time to introduce him to a minute quantity of something new. She found that babies take some time to learn how to digest their first food – their mother's milk – perfectly. After a time, varying between two and a half weeks and three months or more, they give signs of having become 'established' on the breast. These might be a regular gain in weight, sound sleep, a serenity when awake, the beginnings of interest in their surroundings, and faeces of a consistently smooth and creamy texture, mustard yellow in colour, pleasant-smelling and passed at regular – and sometimes long – intervals (even as long as a week) showing that they are digesting their food with efficiency and economy.* (In my limited experience, neither doctors, hospital nurses nor health visitors are interested in the information and help that can be obtained from observation of a baby's stools. It is perhaps noteworthy that in the 1930s and 1940s, 'three months colic' was not the common phenomenon that it is today.) Dr Pearse advocated introducing the baby to new items of food one by one, at intervals of a few days, in order to observe how well he is digesting them; the stools should, of course, change in texture and colour little by little but not too drastically.

Secondly, as I have described in a previous chapter, knowledge of baby-rearing techniques was available to inexperienced parents through the baby clinic, the nursery and through friendly relationships with other young parents and their babies.

A third reason for the development of the faculty for nurture in Centre parents was that, through their use of the Centre, they tended to become 'nourishing' people, or more so than they had been before; their horizons widened, and potential powers and talents hitherto dormant became actual. As Dr W D Wall remarked during his presidential address to the 1970 national conference of the Pre-School Playgroups Association, 'Children grow well when their parents are growing well.' Innes Pearse wrote:

> The gardener can but add elements to the soil, he cannot cause the plant to absorb these elements. So likewise in the nurture of the child we can give nothing; all we can do is to see that we tend the soil and are putting into it the necessary quantity and variety of elements. The old outlook, therefore, must be reviewed. The focus of the parents' attention must be shifted from concentration on what they will give the child, to concentration on their own lives. It is only by their own development, physical and mental, that they can enrich the home, and it is the home ultimately which is the child's environment. This is the soil in which the human seedling must grow.†

The interests, occupations and skills of parents, the decisions they make together, their expressed thoughts and feelings, the stories they tell, the friends they bring into the house or visit, their relationships with their neighbours and the tasks they undertake for the joy of it or for the sake of neighbours, friends and relatives or the community in general – all these bring the world into the home and feed the fire of the child's curiosity about, and love for, what is not itself.

It turned out that young parents found it advantageous to have made good use of the Centre for a short time before becoming parents. Apart from having had time to have any physiological deficiencies or disorders rectified, and having enjoyed varied exercise for their bodies and minds, they had made acquaintances, some of whom were ready to share their joy in becoming parents. It was to be expected that when a new baby

* 1943, p. 171
† 1926

was brought into the cafeteria or the Long Room, many people would come to look and admire, but some of the parents' new acquaintances would share with them a lasting joy in the addition to the family, and this cemented friendships.

It is, I think, a fact that most parents feel wonder – if only for a fleeting moment – at the marvellous ability of a baby to grow in capability as well as in size and strength. For some Centre parents, conversations with the Biologists and observation of other people's babies had the effect of extending these moments of reverence for life, until they grew into an abiding respect for the biological wisdom of their child – and of all children. Another effect was the growth of appreciation of the unique personality of each baby, for as they became acquainted with each other's babies, they could hardly avoid noticing how different each was in feature, physique, temperament, interests and other characteristics. Few Peckham parents at that time were in the habit of reading manuals on how the 'normal' baby should behave or at what age it should be capable of doing this, that or the other. I got the impression that there was little of the worry or envy that can be caused by measuring and comparing one's own baby's progress with that of others: parents' enjoyment, interest and amusement were relatively unalloyed.

Also faith in their own powers grew; they realised that it is not necessary to be a professional or highly educated person to understand about nurture. The desire of a large group of parents to be responsible for the running of an Infant School in the Centre was evidence of this. As I have related, families were discussing this project before the war, and they brought the subject up again soon after the post-war reopening, at a time when the Biologists themselves were so much occupied with the problems of re-equipment and restaffing that they would have preferred to postpone it a little.

As is described in *The Peckham Experiment*, the social life and outside activities of young couples in Peckham at that time often stopped abruptly on the birth of their first child. For Centre members, this did not happen. After a few weeks, when the baby had ceased to be quite so new and mysterious, they brought it sometimes to the night nursery, or came to the Centre in the afternoons, and took up their interrupted social activities. Mothers had no need to be confined all day to the company of a toddler or two, as continued so often to be the case in this country (except for those who could afford nursemaids or those who opted for work outside the home and the use of a child minder or day nursery) until, in 1960, the Pre-School Playgroups Association was founded and community playgroups and mother and toddler clubs began to mushroom. At the Centre, parents could continue to grow – to become 'nourishing' people. The children left in the nursery did not appear to miss their mothers after they had discovered that it was a very good place in which to play. The mothers were free to have an hour or two to themselves and to obtain the stimulation and refreshment of adult company. If they were worried about their children, they could peep at them through the glass doors of the nursery or, of course, fetch them out and bring them into one of the main lounges to sit in their laps for a little.

The pleasure of parents at the discovery that parenthood could be a far more rewarding state than they had previously found it to be, communicated itself, through the convivial atmosphere of the Centre, to younger members. Newly-weds looked forward with confidence to the arrival of their first-born; they realised that the arrival of a child need not cause their lives to be constricted or their relationship to disintegrate. More than half the babies conceived during the families' membership of the Centre were known to be planned.

Expectant mothers who were blooming and full of energy up to the moment of delivery were common, and 85 per cent of babies were breast-fed up to the time when they were weaned on to solids and could drink from a cup. It was well known to Centre members that 'Centre babies' were usually lively and contented and free of ailments; sentiments such as 'it's no trouble to have a baby here' were often expressed. They even attributed qualities of character and temperament in their children to the fact that their earlier years had been spent in the Centre. The letter quoted previously that Gladys and Harry Coring wrote to the Doctors in 1950 included the following:

> Alan took quite a while to settle, now he has taught himself to swim, play billiards, and he has a mind of his own in all things.
>
> When we joined the Centre, Joy was eighteen months old, not physically strong, which had an influence on her general development. Now she is a school girl with an individual personality all her own, and her health has improved to such standards as I would never have believed possible.
>
> Now Valerie of the three children is a Centre baby – I could not have wished for a more natural child, she seemed to know her way in life from the very beginning, and nothing could shake her from that course – strangers have picked her out from a group for her personality, and her ability to know what she wants and get it.

The gratitude to the Centre doctors felt by so many of the members was, I believe, quite often inspired by the help they had received from them in the form of information on the healthy rearing of children. Family consultations before and after the birth of a child and during its early development were much in demand and the doctor conducting the baby clinic was always busy.

Nevertheless, at the time I was planning this book and re-reading all the PHC literature, I felt embarrassed by the impression sometimes given by Innes Pearse of an intention to teach the members how to live. I felt this was at variance with the purpose of the experiment, and I was worried by the thought that people might get the false impression that the Centre staff were occupied in looking for opportunities to give what is called 'health education'. Further thought has led me to the conclusion that Dr Pearse was justified in her efforts to get over to the families her views on good child-rearing practices and to stress the importance of whole, unprocessed and fresh food during pregnancy and lactation. My change of mind is due in the main to a realisation of the fact that, although people's desire to nurture their children to the best of their ability is surely instinctive, the knowledge of how best to go about it is probably not. I have noticed that students of primate behaviour have produced evidence that points to the likelihood of skill in mothering being culture-induced. Gorillas are animals with many similarities to man but one would expect them to be far more governed by instinct, yet John Aspinall, talking in a television programme about gorillas, reported that the two or three infants born in his imaginatively appointed zoo have all had to be taken away from their mothers and reared by the attendants, because the mothers, themselves captured in infancy, had no idea how to care for their babies. He surmised that these gorilla mothers had missed out on the experience, usual for gorillas in the wild, of growing up in family groups containing several mothers and their young of various ages. Dr Harry Harlow found that female rhesus monkeys, separated at birth from their mothers and reared to puberty in groups of four to a cage and then released on to an island inhabited by a troupe of wild monkeys, proved to be bad mothers themselves.[*] Drs Diane Fossey and Jane Goodall who each spent fifteen years or more studying, respectively, gorillas and chimpanzees in the wild, both observed that young female animals are insatiably curious about new-born babies and that they will follow a mother with a new baby about, and squat close to her, waiting for an opportunity to see, touch and, eventually, play with the baby. Perhaps they have an instinct to learn the skill of mothering. A similar attraction to babies can be observed in little girls and sometimes in boys too. But nowadays children and adolescents rarely have the opportunity to satisfy any desire they may have to learn the art of mothering; and many a young mother may never have held a baby in her arms until she finds herself in sole charge of her own. The lack of confidence she feels must be very frightening. Mrs Ethelyn Hazell, who joined six weeks affter her baby was born, recalled how she had felt when she left the maternity hospital:

> I was terrified at being landed with a baby, felt I would not be any good
> as a mother, wished I had not taken it on and hadn't a clue what to do.

If she had joined a few months earlier, she would have had the chance to help in the babies' nursery or to hold and handle the babies of acquaintances and learn useful tips from the mothers. The baby may be

[*] 1962

frightened too. Surely, it may make quite a difference to the way in which a baby views the world, if its mother is not suffering too badly from beginner's nerves the first time she handles it.

Innes Pearse did not lecture the parents, but I think she left them in no doubt of her opinions. Elsie Purser has mentioned her dislike of waterproof pants for babies, because of the danger of sore and inflamed bottoms. Not all mothers dispensed with them entirely as a result: I have heard that a whipping off of the offending garment was frequently to be seen in the waiting room.

The two doctors were complementary personalities. Without the unique characteristics, abilities and talents of each, the Centre would never have materialised. One of the differences between them was that Innes Pearse had much more of the teacher in her make-up. Scott Williamson was, above all, a scientist. His overriding aim was to form, test and develop hypotheses of the nature of health and of basic human needs. He was absolutely consistent in his determination not to influence members' decisions or choices, and not to attempt to *persuade* them to behave in ways that might improve their health. At the same time he fully agreed with Innes Pearse that in order to have a good chance of positive health, a person needs a favourable beginning to his life; and he knew that the implementation of his theories would be much more likely to be successful in bringing about a healthy society in the Centre, and in future Centres elsewhere, if the nurture of the babies, who would eventually people these Centres, were to be of the kind needed by babies. Amy Moor, the Biologists' receptionist and a dedicated and indispensable member of the Centre staff from the beginning, always ready to take on any necessary job, has told me that, on one occasion, she and Scott Williamson were watching the activity in the pool. A young couple were playing in the water with their laughing baby. After a little while, the wife took the baby and disappeared down the steps to the changing room. Apparently she dried it and handed it to the nursery nurse through the door of the changing room that communicated with the nursery, for she returned in a few minutes to rejoin her husband in the pool. Scott Williamson said, 'That's what I am trying to do. Your aches and pains I can alleviate but it's the next generation that I hope to help to lead a fuller life.' So there is no doubt that he sympathised with Innes Pearse's burning desire to pass on to the Centre parents the knowledge she had acquired in her special field of interest, and to help them to rear superbly healthy and happy babies and to enjoy being parents as a result.

As Dr Pearse has related, she relied as much as possible on what she called 'gossip' to spread the information she wished to share with parents. Certainly, the babies planned and conceived after their parents had joined the Centre acted as powerful advertisements for her baby-care methods and her understanding of the needs of pregnant women.

Dr John Ashton, although he had never seen the Centre in action, wrote an extremely perceptive, short but meaty article on the Centre.* He realised that the health education obtained by members of the Pioneer Health Centre was self-education. Their interest in health was aroused by their conversations with the Biologists. Then they actively sought the knowledge that would enable them and their children to lead a healthier more rewarding life. And their desire for it was fanned as much by the general effects of membership and by what they saw happening to their children and friends and acquaintances and felt happening to themselves as a result of their use of the Centre, as by their contacts with the Biologists.

The relationship between the Biologists and the member-families had the overall effect of enabling people to trust their own judgement and become aware of their most deep-seated instincts and feelings.

There was yet another way in which membership of the Centre facilitated the development of the faculty for nurture in people. When all the family made use of the Centre, communication between parents and children became easier, for they had a common ground of experience. They might be doing entirely different things in the Centre and hardly see each other while they were in the building or they might be there at different times of the day or the week, but they could talk to each other about their experiences and doings and be understood; they would all know the building well and have watched from time to time the various activities that went on, and they usually knew each other's friends and acquaintances. Moreover since the building was open all the afternoon and evening six days a week, there was usually some time during the week when a father could join the rest of the family in the pool or play a game of billiards or table tennis with his son or daughter. So there were plenty of subjects of conversation at meal times in which all could share. Families usually gathered in their own homes for main meals; dinners were not provided at the cafeteria counter at any time of the day. Snacks were available during the afternoons and light supper dishes in the evening. It happened on several occasions that staff members were told how family mealtimes had become much more lively occasions than they had been before the family joined. One mother remarked, 'The strange thing is that before we joined the Centre we never had anything to talk about at home, and now mealtimes are always a buzz.' This allows one to guess that the atmosphere in these families had become more conducive to the sharing of thoughts and feelings than they had formerly been, so that an individual might find himself describing his experiences to the family and obtaining their aid in the mental digestion of the experiences.

* * * * *

* 1977

I do not claim that the effects of membership described in this section were universal in the Centre. There were a large number of families for which they were true and since the members of these families were often to be seen in the building, the Biologists and their colleagues knew them well. But there were also, at any time, families among the membership who, for various reasons, did not become an integral part of the Centre and did not appreciate its full value, using it merely as a temporary convenience. These families helped to swell the number of those who sooner or later let their membership lapse. There were also some, as I have said earlier, who were unavoidably prevented from using the Centre much, but remained members for the sake of the overhaul and the consultations with the Biologists, or because one or other member of the family particularly appreciated the facilities offered. In some cases, the children made a great deal more use of the Centre than their parents; but, as I remember, the behaviour of most of these children, while they were in the building, was healthy in the Peckham sense of the word.

* * * * *

Being a nurturing parent consists not only in providing an environment in which a child can grow, but also in weaning him from dependence on oneself. One has to let go and allow him to stand on his own two feet and become responsible for himself, in one field of activity after another.

Scott Williamson said that the best place for a seedling tree to grow is at the edge of the shadow cast by the parent tree.

> We regard the function of parenthood as that of weaning the child stage by stage, from the specific parental environment to the general environment of the outer world.*

Weaning is by definition a smooth and gradual process, but not necessarily a slow one. Parents and child both play a part in it. In some fields of activity, a child will want to – and need to – exercise independent judgement and become self-reliant at a very young age, for example, in the field of his movement in relation to the force of gravity; in others, for example, movement in relation to motor traffic, parents will need to keep control until the child has learned how motor vehicles behave and the rules of the road and has acquired the virtue of patience.

Dr Pearse coined the phrase 'skirt weaning' for the gradual growth of the small child's ability to do without the constant company of one or other of its parents. She found instances when this weaning had not occurred and mother and child had become so habituated to each other's presence that any separation was a traumatic experience for both of them. When people lived in less artificial, less man-made surroundings, when families were bigger, and the whole farmstead or small town was 'home' which the child was able to explore little by little as he felt able,

* 1938, p. 46

weaning in this sense would have occurred without anyone being aware of it. Nowadays, even when parents realise the need for it, they find it difficult to prevent their children from being in a state of overclose dependence on themselves for three, four or five years and then suddenly pitchforked into the milling crowd of the school playground or the Day Nursery. They find it impossible to wean their children in an environment composed of supermarkets, streets used by potentially lethal motor traffic, and apartment blocks, where, for various reasons, neighbours are strangers to each other and strangers' children are a nuisance. It may be almost as difficult in suburbs where, because of our aging population, the nearest family of young children may live at some distance.

At the Centre, most families found weaning relatively easy. In many cases the children of school age could come to the Centre on their own, when and if they felt like it. The parents would know where the children were and roughly the sort of thing they would be doing. The children for their part would usually have the opportunity to watch their parents pursuing their chosen interests and forms of relaxation. In this way, the parents' choice might affect the child, but he was free to follow or not to follow in his parents' footsteps. He could strike out in another direction and cultivate his own particular talents and interests; he could, if he wished, try learning several different skills in quick succession without causing worry or arguments in the family or anyone making a big thing of it; or he could just play. Adge Elven recalled suddenly finding himself a member of the swimming team of his school as a result of playing every day in the Centre swimming pool. Each member of the family could enjoy himself according to his taste without getting in the hair of the others or, alternatively, becoming isolated from the others through spending his leisure in places into which they could not easily follow him or know anything about.

At the Centre, children could choose to imitate and learn from other adults than their parents; they could observe the behaviour and learn the opinions of people of all ages and kinds and thus nourish their own power of judgement and discrimination: friendships developed between whole families, and acquaintances were of all ages. For families who made themselves a part of the community of the Centre, there was no generation gap.

For that reason, there should, in theory, have been less friction between adolescents and their parents and more mutual understanding and respect. Recently, I have asked several former members of the Centre to tell me what they felt, in retrospect, was the Centre's greatest single benefit for them. There was a variety of answers. Some said that access to a doctor who was also a friend was the thing they most valued, others the freedom to do what you liked when you liked, or the long-term friendships that they made or the confidence it gave them, but some cited the fact that it was a family club, expressing themselves in such words as, 'It was a place to which all the family liked to go'. Perhaps this last can be taken as evidence that use of the Centre developed independence in the children without at the same time destroying their friendship and unity with their parents. An instance, from the child's angle, of how membership of the Centre assisted the weaning of parent and child from dependence on each other came when a staff member asked a schoolgirl how her mother was, 'Oh, she's fine, thank you. Now she has learned to swim, she does not worry about us all the time.' 'Learning to swim' meant much more than it would have done when used in another context. It meant not only meeting a group of women regularly, but also the opportunity to follow up the acquaintanceship by meeting each other at other times, doing other things together and getting to know each other's families. The daughter's reply suggested not only that her mother was happier since she had learned to swim but also that she herself and her siblings were finding their mother better company. When husband and wife and children were all 'growing', there was an increase in their enjoyment of each other as people. Families tended to become more united as the individuality of each member blossomed. Members were aware of a flowering of their capabilities. 'The Centre', one burly father of teenagers told an interviewer from the BBC, 'fair blossomed me out.'

That weaning, in the sense of the growth of the ability to exercise independent judgement, to think, speak and choose for oneself, continues well into adolescence is, I think, generally agreed. But, so often, it seems to me, the young merely exchange dependence on their parents for dependence on the peer group; they take over quite uncritically the prevailing teenage tastes, and fashions of behaviour. The Peckham Biologists held that the maturing of individuality and responsibility needs a family environment in which to happen – but not a family environment alone. When a family belonged to the Centre, a teenager was able to live at home without experiencing claustrophobia, suffocation or constriction and to suffer little from parental suspicion of his activity outside the home. He could develop his individuality and autonomy to a self-respecting degree, without having to stage repeated revolts or cut his umbilical cord as it were. For his 'home' became something nearer to the meaning given to the word by the Biologists – the 'field of excursion' of the family. To Williamson and Pearse a 'home' is something a family creates that fulfils and expresses its unique individuality; it is a bit of the world that becomes patterned with the particular quality of that family; it extends far beyond the four walls of the house or appartment. As the members of a united and communicating family follow their own particular interests and activities and make their own friends, they each extend and enrich the 'home', the 'home' grows in diversity and individuality through the ever-widening 'functional excursion' of the family.

In a sense, the Centre consisted of the totality of the 'homes' of the member-families. I think it was important that the propinquity of the families was not enforced: they could retire into the privacy of their own houses or apartments at will. But the Centre was a stable whole within which every 'home' could be affected and enriched by every other. When families and individuals live an isolated existence, merely bumping up against an unending crowd of strangers or vaguely recognised faces, their 'homes' cannot be mutually enriching.

Perhaps it was the creative integration of unique 'homes' that caused the particular 'Centre atmosphere' that visitors sometimes felt and re-marked upon. Howard Marshall, the radio commentator, knew the Centre well. He had visited it more than once, in the early days. In 1949, he was the host in Radio Sports Club which was broadcast from the Centre for a period during that year every Tuesday evening, with well-known sports-men as guests. He wrote in the Bulletin of the Pioneer Health Centre of June 1949:

> There is an atmosphere about the Centre which is difficult to define. It was always there, and it remains unchanged. Perhaps those who use the Centre daily are less conscious of it than visitors. It is a sense of independence, of uninhibited and natural behaviour, of individual free-dom, unusual in the ordinary organised community. Possibly this is because the Family Club is not organised, in the usually accepted sense of organisation. Here there is spontaneous growth. The growth of the Centre is organic. It develops like a plant, with living force.

* * * * *

Scott Williamson has been criticised by a social historian for being 'rigid' and 'a dictator'. It is true that he assumed the leadership of the loyal, but not uncritical, executive committee of his supporting body, the Pioneer Health Centre Ltd. It is also true that, towards the end when money was desperately needed, he insisted on carrying on his search into the nature of health in the manner that he had found to be successful so far, rather than accept grants with strings attached or hand over any control to an outside body. Here the members were behind him, as the sequel proved. When the Centre became bankrupt and the building was bought by the London County Council, the Members' Association, for-med to save the Centre, (see Mrs Purser's Experience, Chapter 8) tried to negotiate with them. The LCC intended to separate the infant welfare and ante-natal services, which they categorised as preventive medicine, from the leisure facilities. These they proposed to hand over to the Education Committee of the LCC who planned to turn the main part of the building into an 'Evening Institute'. They told the Members' Association that they could use the preventive medical facilities and the Evening Institute. The Members' Association knew that Evening

Institutes merely provided courses in various skills, some for adults, some for older children, and that it was necessary to sign on for a term (about ten weeks) of weekly sessions. They refused the offer, saying what they wanted was a family club. They said:

> ... a family club should provide equally for all members of the family, and facilities should be such that, while mother and father are engaged in activities or even just having a cup of tea, the children could be there also, each conscious of the other.

From the members' behaviour and remarks at the time and from what they have said since, it is evident that each felt free to use the Centre in his own way and to add his personal contribution to its continuing creation. In fact, some members felt (it was about the only criticism expressed) there should have been more organisation and control by the management. Nothing could have been less dictatorial than Scott Williamson's behaviour towards the members of the Centre. Moreover his opinions and theories were strongly held but not rigidly; he was ready to adapt them when new facts emerged.

The large majority of members – adults and children – showed by their behaviour that they felt it was *their* Centre in spite of the fact that it was also someone else's scientific research establishment. Probably, the knowledge that they were, through the family weekly subscription and the charges paid by adults for the use of any of the facilities, partly financing the Centre, contributed to this feeling; but, more important was their growing awareness that the experiment – the research itself – required that they should be individually their own masters and entirely free to be themselves, short of robbing anyone else of this freedom. Therefore, they were happy to allow Scott Williamson the responsibility for the overall organisation of his research-station-cum-family-club. They trusted him because, as they got to know him, they realised that he was, however warm-hearted, a scientist through and through, an objective seeker after truth and *not* a do-gooder trying in an extra subtle way to mould people into his particular idea of how they should be. Therefore, they did not feel 'got at', and many of them understood and respected his desire that no-one should cause any other member to feel powerless because in a minority.

A respect for individuality and an enjoyment of the diversity of human nature did grow in the Centre, including the mutual respect of the old and the young.

In the space of two or three years, the conditions instituted and maintained by Scott Williamson and his team enabled the creation, by the member families – *not* by Scott Williamson and his team – of an enduring neighbourhood community.

Chapter 6

The Financial Failure

This chapter is something of a digression. I have included it because people so often ask the question, 'Why did the Centre fail?'

The short answer is that the Centre did *not* fail; it ran out of money, but not before it had yielded valuable information concerning the nature and needs of humankind.

As may already be evident to the reader, it was a success from many points of view:

1. It was a piece of observational research in the field of human ethology, a field that had not been explored before – and very little since – because of the difficulty of observing humans 'in the wild'.

2. The long-term member-families were very sure of its success as a social experiment, and as a place where people could improve their health and that of their children.

3. To Scott Williamson and Innes Pearse and their colleagues, the vitality, spontaneity, and responsibility of the members, and the harmony and diversity in the community life of the Centre was evidence that they were on the right road towards the discovery of circumstances in which people's health can blossom.

The 1938 report – *Biologists in Search of Material* – created a sensation because of the evidence it gave of the nation's poor state of health, but some people were aware of its deeper message and welcomed it with enthusiasm. John Hilton, Professor of Industrial Relations in Cambridge wrote in the *News Chronicle*:

> There at Peckham, it seems to me, is being discovered by first-hand observation, the basic laws of healthy and happy and abundant living.

Dr Ernest Barker, Professor of Political Science, Cambridge, wrote in *The Observer*:

> This is a pamphlet of a hundred pages which is enough to set every reader thinking – thinking, wondering and hoping.

The Scientific Correspondent of *The Manchester Guardian* wrote:

> The Peckham investigators have collected some very interesting observations... It is to be hoped that their unique attempt to discover the nature

of positively healthy living, as distinct from cures for disease, will receive adequate financial support.

Hamilton Fyfe wrote in *Reynold's News*:

So clearly a national health service ought to include centres of this kind for everybody. The money spent on them would be saved in other ways.

And the *Sunday Times* published a long appreciation of the report by Professor R G Stapledon called *Tracing New Paths in Biology – Pioneer Work of a Health Centre*. This includes:

Having myself conducted prolonged researches on plant communities, I believe I am by that much better equipped to appreciate the immense importance to mankind of the researches of Drs Williamson and Pearse and their colleagues at the Pioneer Health Centre in Peckham.

What chiefly impresses the biologist reading this report is that here, and almost for the first time, we see biology being definitely applied to the service of man, and that we are given a clear lead as to what should be the legitimate aims of biology, what are, in fact, and by right, its material and methods and the form its technology should take.

...The supreme teaching of the Peckham researches is that 'Nature is that which we obey.' Only at his peril can man ignore his own biological limitations: man needs must study himself, and with a degree of intensity in exact proportion to the advances made by all the other sciences. It follows therefore that the conduct of researches which must inevitably lead towards a more general recognition of this sadly neglected truth constitutes a pioneer service of inestimable value to mankind.'

Then, in 1943, *The Peckham Experiment* was published. It sold 50,000 copies in five years. The experiment became famous. During the last eighteen months of its existence, it was visited by 12,000 people from all over the country and the world. The hard-pressed staff found themselves spending more time than they could spare from their work showing visitors around and wearing themselves out travelling in order to give talks to the organisations requesting them. Press opinions of *The Peckham Experiment* included:

This book is so full of meat and so brilliant, both analytically and synthetically, that subtle and thought-stimulating quotations might be taken from every page... among the most important sociological work... that has appeared in the last decade.

The Times Educational Supplement

This fascinating and extremely important book describes the growth of the experiment; the spontaneous integration of over a thousand families into a living social group; the organic structure of that group; and the conclusions drawn by observers, thrilling in terms of their own anthropological, biological and medical training.

Time and Tide

Much can be learned from this great experiment. Let us hope that it will be multiplied a thousandfold after the war and form a cornerstone in the construction of the national health service.

Industrial Welfare

Lord Geddes, GCMG, KCB, MD wrote:

Here at Peckham, in this Pioneer Health Centre, you have the first conscious attempt to create and enrich the social environment so necessary if young married couples are to mature. Here, the need of easy social contacts, if health and well-being are to be attained, is firmly grasped and understood. As I have studied the reports of the work done here, I have come to realise the full meaning of the social elements in that wholeness which is positive health.

and Herbert Read:

It is a great experiment, with far-reaching consequences in politics and sociology... The book is not only fascinating reading: it embodies valuable scientific investigation and will undoubtedly be regarded as a classic in those future days when the biological conception of human society is more fully appreciated.

In 1950, in a letter to *The Times*, Sir C Stanton Hicks, Professor of Human Physiology and Pharmacology, University of Adelaide, wrote:

Sir, – The distressing news has reached Australia that the Pioneer Health Centre is in financial straits likely indeed to bring its short though epoch-making life to an ignominious close. Ignominious because the Peckham Experiment in human biology marks the first attempt successfully to evaluate the effect of the various factors that combine to influence the health of human family groups in this modern age, and because it is so typically British in its practical approach.

If changing circumstance is so profoundly to undermine this capacity of the mother country to provide such fruitful evidence of independent intellectual leadership as is amply demonstrated in the Peckham Experiment, then indeed will the future for our influence in human affairs be in decline.

In times when the emphasis upon disease and its treatment has reached such a stage that the national expenditure upon ill-health has already assumed proportions which embarrass the Treasury, surely knowledge of the essentials of health are greater than ever before? This is just what the Peckham Experiment continues to provide at a cost which is infinitesimal by comparison, and the results of the application of which would brighten the lives of men and reduce the colossal burden on the taxpayer.

It is not too late to stop this trend, and only Britain has demonstrated through the Peckham Experiment the way of escape. The mother country has not failed in immeasurably more hazardous and costly enterprises to set an example to her overseas children. Let us hope that she will not do so on this vital instance of the Peckham Experiment.

I am, yours sincerely, C. STANTON HICKS

What failed to occur was the realisation of the founders' hope that, after an initial experimental and stabilising period, the Centre would be self-supporting. As I have noted, it was, to Scott Williamson, one of the essential environmental conditions of the experiment that the member-families should be as much as possible financially responsible for their family health club, for he held that responsibility for oneself and one's circumstances is a necessary component of health, and, therefore, a health-promoting environment must provide the opportunity for the exercise of responsibility. For this reason, it was important to the Biologists that the financial contributions of the members should cover the running costs of the Centre including the salaries of all the staff. Because this did not come about, it should not be inferred that the Centre was a failure as a social institution any more than as a research under-taking. Users' fees, in spite of being high, cover only a tiny fraction of the running costs of the modern urban 'leisure centres' which are almost entirely financed from rates and taxes. These centres provide extensive indoor sports and recreational facilities and are open to all who can afford to pay. In the case of a very spacious and well appointed leisure centre in the north of London, I was told that very few of the inhabitants of the area could afford to use it. Unlike the Pioneer Health Centre, these centres do not provide the circumstances in which a neighbourhood community can grow and flourish.

Before building was begun on the St Mary's Road site, it had been calculated that income from the weekly family subscriptions and from charges made for the use of recreational facilities would cover running costs, as soon as the membership reached 1,700 to 2,000 families. From the experience of the pilot scheme in 1926–9, it was judged that this number would be reached three years after opening. In fact, a member-ship of this size was never achieved.

Of the families who joined after the war, at least 50 per cent sooner or later dropped out. No records were kept of the reasons for leaving and no member of staff could be spared to chase the families who were falling behind with their subscriptions. At the outbreak of war in Sep-tember 1939, there were 875 paid-up member-families; this number was never exceeded.

It will be recalled that the Biologists hoped that the membership would represent all income groups. This proved to be the case; in 1938, members' incomes ranged from £2:5s to £20 a week. Harry and Gladys Coring joined soon after the post-war reopening. Harry recalled, many years later, of his Centre companions:

We were a mixed lot, from lawyers to dustmen. I remember a builder – quite well off, a shirt cutter, a doctor, a printer. Members got together because they enjoyed doing similar things.

Some members considered the subscription absurdly low; it was kept low so as not to exclude any families living in the Centre 'District' (the area around the Centre from which families were eligible for membership) who wanted to join. In fact a large number of families at the lower end of the scale paid up regularly for years. The Corings' income at that time was very low. Gladys said:

In those days, you could go to the pictures for two shillings and six-pence* – two of you. So I thought about it in those terms – it will mean giving up the pictures. We never went to the pictures after we joined.

One reason for the high turnover of members was the condition of the housing in the area. This looked consistently respectable from the outside but in many streets was overcrowded and seriously lacking in mod cons. There was a preponderance of originally middle-class Victorian and Edwardian terrace houses, some still occupied by one family but mostly by two, three or more families sharing exiguous toilet facilities and with makeshift kitchens. In some of these houses, the only running water available was on the ground floor, and the only WC was outside, reached through the kitchen of the people occupying the ground floor. The unsatisfactory housing caused much movement in and out of the area.

After the war, the housing situation was still worse. Bombing of the nearby docks had caused extensive damage, and the houses that remained intact had deteriorated through neglect. It was a measure of the value of the Centre to its members that so many of them remained in the Centre 'District' or chose to return to it when the war was over.

In general, during the war years, there had been a change in people's expectations. Families who had cheerfully accepted shared front doors and toilets and no bathroom, now felt that a post-war 'prefab' was preferable, and went in search of one. Some Centre families found one outside the 'District' and were permitted to remain members although they may have used the Centre less frequently as a result. The shortage of houses was so great that families were living in rooms requisitioned by the Local Authority in other families' houses, often against the will of the latter.

So, the area ceased to attract a stable population of sufficient size to support a Centre financially. If war had not intervened, it is possible that the membership would have continued to rise slowly but steadily as it had done up to the summer of 1939.

Today, Peckham would not be a place in which to try to set up a PHC. Rita Herron, whose family were members during her childhood and who organises play schemes for the local education authority tells

* 30 old pence

me, 'Half the school population changes every year: the mobility is unbelievable.'

It was found, before the war, that there was, in the area, a surprising lack of friendly contact between neighbours. Indeed, it often happened that a family made friends with a neighbouring family only after they had both joined the Centre. The fact that people were often hoping to move to a better apartment and in the meantime jealously guarded what little privacy they had, may have contributed to the lack of acquaintance between neighbours, and this in turn may have been one of the causes of the slow growth of membership.

Today, few people would, I think, be deterred by the idea of a medical examination but at that period some people, especially men, were shy of it. Mrs Coring recalled, 'I didn't worry about the medical after having had children... the thought of it might have deterred me before I had had babies.'

Many middle-aged or elderly couples found membership worthwhile, and widows or widowers whose children had taken up family membership found it a godsend, for it enabled them to share in the life of the younger family without intruding into the privacy of their home. Nevertheless, the Centre was, to start with, attractive mainly to families with babies, or children still at school. This set a limit to the number of families likely to join, during the Centre's first years, from among the population of 5,500 households living in the Centre 'District'.

It will be remembered that it was necessary for the purposes of the experiment to offer membership only to the families living within easy and safe walking distance of the Centre building. On three sides, the boundary of the 'District' followed in the main the physical boundaries formed by railway lines. This part of London is covered not by a network so much as a crochetwork of railway lines. These originally joined villages and suburbs but were built earlier than the main mass of houses and were infrequently bridged. The fourth boundary followed a road which was one of the main thoroughfares from central London into southern Kent and East Sussex. The Centre was close to this road, so the 'District' was shaped more like a semicircle than a circle. In 1937 it was decided to enlarge the 'District' by taking in an area on the far side of the main road. Some families in this area had been longing to join and, for a time, there was a considerable increase in the number of enrolments, but in the long-term the increase in the membership was not proportionate to the increase in the size of the 'District'.

So it turned out that the Centre's annual income was considerably less than had been estimated. Expenditure proved to be slightly greater than had been expected. The building had not been expensive to build; it had cost (in 1935) £38,000, including basic equipment, but heating costs were high. The generous donations made by private individuals were swallowed up and solvency was only restored during the war when the building was let for industrial use. After the war, the Sir Halley Stewart Trust offered a grant on condition that the Centre open immediately, but much of this was inevitably used for the almost total re-equipment that was necessary, and appeals to the public for financial support were not sufficiently successful. Why was this? Here are some probable reasons that occur to me.

1. Many of the hundreds of visitors who made their way to Peckham during the Centre's last years expressed a great desire to have similar Centres in their own areas but were not prepared to contribute much to the expenses of the prototype. This was a time when people were working hard to rebuild their own lives after the upheavals and depredations of the war.

2. It was not the kind of cause that tugs at people's heartstrings as do appeals for the starving, the disabled, abused children or cancer research. Moreover it was impossible to get the purpose of the Centre across in the space of an advertisement or radio appeal: its scope was too comprehensive.

3. At the time, people in general tended to agree with Sir William Beveridge that the nation's health would be assured if everyone were guaranteed an income sufficient for food, clothing and shelter, free education and a free and comprehensive medical service. At that time, faith and hope were centred on the Welfare State.

No support was forthcoming from national or local government. At the time, the government departments responsible for health and social services were occupied with the inauguration of the new National Health Service. They held that the Pioneer Health Centre could not be fitted into the NHS because it was not open to everybody wherever they might live, but only to local families, and because it was not free but required a subscription-paying membership.

I think it can be said that in general, at this period, public taste was for more government, for centralised planning and organisation and for equality even at the expense of freedom and creativity. The politicians of the time were following the majority will. But it is possible that the attitude of members of government bodies to the Centre was influenced by a desire – common in people in positions of authority – that those in their charge should be easy to lead and control. This tendency can be observed in such parents as invariably use the adjective 'independent' in a pejorative sense when describing their young children. Several members of the Centre staff remember noticing a marked lack of sympathy with the theory and practice of the Centre in some of those visitors to the centre who were employed in administrative and official positions. They seemed to be prejudiced against it. Perhaps it was the members' outspoken independence of mind and obvious enjoyment of the exercise of individual autonomy that worried them. Perhaps they had a lurking distrust of something that might cause people's behaviour to become less predictable.

The desire for equality at all costs contributed to the tragic fate of the brave attempt by a group of people in Coventry at the end of the war to set up a Centre modelled on the PHC. During the war the group formed the Family Health Club Housing Association and, when their numbers reached 350 families, bought 300 acres of land on the edge of Coventry – an industrial city seriously short of houses. As Dr Kenneth Barlow writes:

> Instead of the environment being set up and people being fitted into it, on this occasion, people were to assemble and to make their environment fit their biological needs.*

Their plans for 2,000 houses and neighbourhood amenities, including schools, a Peckham-type Centre and a small farm, were accepted by the Warwickshire County Council. They expected to be able to go ahead as soon as peace was restored. But in the event, the new Town and Country Planning Act put an end to private building for many years, the Ministry of Health, concentrating on the treatment of the sick, had no funds available for the promotion of health, and the Coventry City Council opposed the scheme on the grounds that no group should be encouraged to have what was not available to everyone. No licence to build was forthcoming. To be strictly accurate, the Family Health Club Housing Association was granted a licence to build two houses a year!

Although at the time there were individuals on both sides of both Houses of Parliament who appreciated the value of the PHC, I doubt if the leadership as a whole of any party would have welcomed the prospect of Centres of the Peckham kind spreading over the whole country.

Of late, there has been a change of attitude. A person is less ready to believe that members of governments, officials, specialists or senior academics know better than he does himself what his and his children's needs are and how he should behave. Equality of opportunity is as much desired as ever, but freedom of choice and action and personal responsibility for the course of one's own life are also ardently sought by many people.

The lack of government approval at this period was a deterrent to the charitable trusts and foundations both in this country and abroad – apart from the Sir Halley Stewart Trust. The director of one big American foundation, to which an appeal was made, wrote that their policy was to refrain from supporting any venture that appeared to be contrary to the policy of the government of the country concerned.

* 1988

Finally, there was a complete failure on the part of the scientific establishment to see that the Centre offered a ready-made opportunity to observe and describe the spontaneous behaviour of relatively healthy people in a relatively healthy social and physical environment. The knowledge of the nature of other species that has been obtained by zoologists prepared to live for years at a time close to wild animals in their natural habitat, watching and noting, was still to come, and so perhaps leaders of the Life Sciences in the 1940s cannot be blamed for failing to realise that comparable observational research was being done on human subjects at the Peckham Centre. Today no-one can deny that our ignorance of the way individual jackdaws, wolves, gorillas and hundreds of other creatures behave in relation to their own kind and to other species, organise their societies and develop their potential capability to the full is well on the way to being dispelled by the methods of observational research – what Niko Tinbergen called 'the basic scientific method of watching and wondering'.*

At that time there were few students of the Life Sciences who were aware of the need to learn about the tendencies, powers, limitations and environmental needs that everyone has because they are human. Most regarded the Peckham Experiment as an interesting luxury. They did not see it as an urgent necessity, providing knowledge that could ensure the survival of our civilisation.

In the field of human ethology and ecology, Scott Williamson was half a century ahead of his time. Even now there is no appreciable response to Tinbergen's call for co-operation in building a 'coherent comprehensive Science of Man'.

One can guess at a further reason why psychologists and sociologists ignored the existence of the Peckham Experiment. In order to obtain for psychology and sociology the status of sciences, they deemed it necessary to confine themselves to research involving the mathematical methods of the 'exact' sciences. For that kind of research, the controlled and limited environment of a laboratory is needed or the use of questionnaires designed to make the results quantifiable. This kind of research can only supply rather minor and superficial items of knowledge. If human ethologists are going to learn about man's true nature, they must unobtrusively observe people in the kind of environment that permits their true nature to develop. Moreover, they must be aware of the uniqueness, the special quality of every person.

Sad to say, the present-day student of the Life Sciences still confines himself to collecting information that can be quantified – reams and reams of it. About eight years ago, a young, enterprising and successful member of a university department of psychology wrote to me:

> There is no escape from the need to measure complex and subtle phenomena... to think how one might quantify, for example, wholeness, spontaneity, individuality, capability for nurture, responsibility.

* 1972

This attitude is deeply engrained in universities. Only very rarely is an individual free of it.

In 1978, two clear-sighted and independent-minded anthropologists, Stephen Boyden and Sheelagh Miller, wrote:

> Our academic institutions are in a position to make a vitally important contribution to the problems of the modern world by improving the holistic understanding of human situations and by encouraging a sense of perspective in human affairs. Unfortunately, however they are at present possessed of a number of characteristics which tend to interfere with their capacity to play this role... One of these is a state of mind which has been called 'quantophrenia', that is – an obsession with numbers. This weakness is closely related, of course, to the preoccupation of society as a whole with the easily measurable aspects of situations. There is, however, no law of nature or of society to the effect that there is likely to be any relationship in human affairs between quantifiability and performance. Consequently, attempts to understand social and societal problems which neglect the relevant unmeasurable and intangible aspects of reality are likely to result in a distorted and unbalanced picture. Needless to say, if pertinent variables can be meaningfully expressed in a quantitative way, then it makes good sense to do so. But when intangible ingredients of dynamic human situations are deemed important on the basis of biosocial principles or even intuition, then we must deal with them in the best way we can, relying on our powers of observation, critical thinking, intelligence and judgement rather than on our computers. It is preferable to do this than to try to put numbers on aspects of human experience which are simply not quantifiable – a practice which can lead to a false sense of security and a dangerous and misplaced sense of accuracy and meaning.*

Mary Midgley writes:

> We need to study people qualitatively as well as quantitatively, individually as well as statistically, in natural conditions as well as experimentally. For these purposes we need to use ordinary observations of the kind we can all make.†

And she quotes Aristotle (*Ethics* 1.3):

> It is the mark of an educated man to look for just as much precision in each enquiry as the nature of the subject allows.

But this is very recent thinking. In the late 1940s no scientist able to command funds for research recognised the unique opportunity afforded by the Pioneer Health Centre to discover important human needs and potentialities and to begin to build a soundly based Science of Man. And Scott Williamson's efforts to convince the scientific establishment that the study of health forces one to consider unquantifiable factors, and that these must be brought into the field of science, failed to make any impression.

* 1978
† 1979

It was to be expected that the Medical Research Council would be more interested in discovering more effective ways of combatting disease than in learning what kind of an environment people need if they are to be healthy. At that time, they were also unable to see the value of research findings that were not reducible to figures. The Council had, for many years, devoted itself to the promotion of the science of epidemiology, which was concerned with the extent and variability of disease among different populations. Sir Austin Bradford Hill, who has been called 'the father of statistics', was one of the most influential members of the MRC, largely because of his work in epidemiology. He visited the Centre, but found nothing there to interest him; he saw that it was unlikely to produce statistics that could contribute to epidemiology. As to research, he was interested only in results drawn from comparisons between groups, one group being a 'control' group from whom treatment or opportunities were withheld. And it must have been as obvious to him as to anyone else, that it was not a place in which research methods of this kind could be used. For him and Scott Williamson, there was no meeting of minds; his was not open to the idea that people are unique, whole and constantly growing organisms of whom no significant knowledge can be obtained by means of statistics or narrowly angled experiments; he completely failed to understand what the Peckham Biologists were trying to do. The MRC decided not to support the Centre or recommend financial assistance. Not only were the charitable trusts influenced by their attitude but, when Aneuran Bevan consulted them as to the possible value of the work being done there for the new National Health Service, they turned down their thumbs.

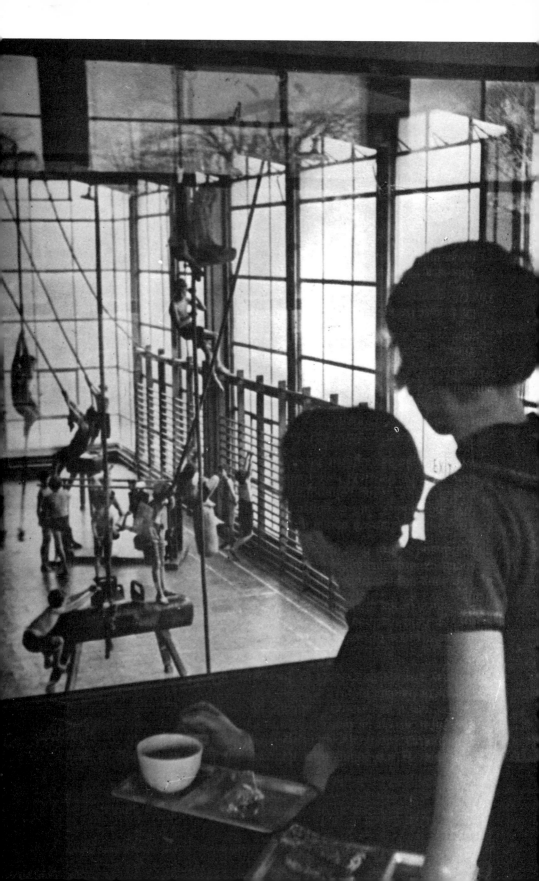

Part Two

Members' Memories

Chapter 7

Excerpts from Conversations with Former Members

Between 1978 and 1985 some former members of the Centre were located and interviewed. With most of them, the Biologists and their staff had had no contact since 1950. From tape recordings of long, rambling and enjoyable conversations, I have extracted the following quite unedited passages. It took some time for people to cast their thoughts back to those far off years. Some confused their memories of the 1935–9 period with those of the 1946–50 period but, as we sat and discussed the state of the world then and now, memories of people, incidents and feelings rose to the surface. Some subsequently wrote letters from which I have quoted.

Olive and John Smith, Sydney, Australia [They emigrated after the Centre closed. John is a Senior Principal Research Scientist in CSIRO. Olive, née Fee, was for many years head of a large state nursery school. She now works with old people.]

John   My parents joined at the beginning – in 1935. I was ten. I remember there was a gymnastics teacher, Mr Peasnell. He conducted classes in the gym; these were utterly boring. This phase of gymnastic activity was short-lived as the kids stopped attending the classes. We were taught breast stroke in strictly controlled classes. The kids who made most progress did so by watching the bigger boys; I know I always closely observed Ron Moody and George Goldstone. There was a bit of ground on two sides of the building. We used to play croquet at the beginning; it was a grassed area then; later it was covered with tarmac. A Miss Coupe used to help us. We used the Centre tools. Mr Peasnell organised the digging of a running track around the perimeter; we dug a deep trench. On a Saturday afternoon, there would be a whole lot of boys digging. It was never finished, but we used to have camps there; in some places the ditch was three or four feet deep and we only had to put a sheet of old corrugated iron over it and we had a hideout. We used to make fires and cook sausages and have a bit of inter-gang warfare – whether the staff knew or not, no-one was concerned. We did just the ordinary things that boys do. But it was the only place in the area where you could do it. Later, when they had the camping at Sissinghurst, my mother took us, my sister and me, camping. My father was dead by then. She used to sleep in the oast house, but we slept in a tent. There was a lake and a rowing boat and we swam. And fishing – I learned to fish there.

When I went to High School, I usually did my home-work at home first, and then spend the rest of the evening at the Centre. I spent all the time I could there. My mother used it a lot. I remember she was in a Gilbert and Sullivan Opera, *Trial by Jury*, that was performed there. I did everything there was to do; I can't think of anything I did not do. My friends did a lot of different things too.

My father was a tram driver. I remember he earned £3:12s a week. After the war, I was at college, but I still used the Centre. I was in the college swimming team, but I brought them to swim against a Centre team. I played in the Centre Dance Band. I did join a jazz band outside – in Wimbledon.

I certainly did not grow out of it. Here, there are lots of sports, soccer, rugby clubs and so on, but the boys begin to drop out at 14. The drop-out rate is remarkable; by 18 there are hardly any left... At the Centre, you learned to do your own thing, and not to resent other people wanting to do their own thing. I would never have met and talked to so many different kinds of people any-where else; there was so much mixing of people.

Olive   Doc made everybody feel they were interesting to him. He had the power to make people feel – whatever they were, garbage dustmen, bank managers, no matter who they were – they were equally important. And he never put on side with anybody. Also he never urged anybody to do anything. Once we were having supper in the Cafe-teria, when I was on the staff. There was a visitor there. Somebody mentioned a man who didn't ever seem to do anything but just sat around. Doc said, 'He has a most dreadful hernia.' The visitor said, 'Why don't you treat it?' Doc said, 'It's his hernia. Its up to him when he wants to get it fixed up.'

I think all the members loved Doc.

My father used the Centre a certain amount. He was a printer and had difficult hours. My mother never used it. I went every day as a child. We joined when I was 11, so I was there between 11 and 15. I remember doing a variety of things, a lot of playing in the gym – I can remember five girls of my age with whom I played most evenings – and in the pool, and especially Saturday afternoons when the gym was crowded with boys and girls of all ages. My friends and I played a lot of badminton, and later we did a lot of dancing too. Then, after the war, I was on the staff. I helped in the nursery and then with the school, and, in the afternoons, I was on the social floor giving out tickets to the children, also bikes and skates, looking after the equipment, and generally supervising the children, and, of course, helping with visitors.

John   There was no way we would have come to Australia if the Centre had remained open. We would never even have thought of it. I had a good job. We were married and had Johnny. We left because life was so empty; there was nothing to do, and nothing ever changed. If the Centre had stayed, there would always have been lots to do. [In Australia, they designed their own house and built it almost all with their own hands in their free time.] Now, I realise, I would not have done so well career-wise in England – my background and accent would have been against me.

      The Centre taught me how to get on with people – and how to leave them free. Scientists must be left free if they are to be creative. I was able to make use of Williamson's philosophy in my work.

Olive   The children at the Centre were definitely not competitive. The parents were not either.

John   I think working class people did not compete with each other in those days; not in our street anyway. Perhaps higher up the hill the attitude was a little different.

Olive   I think they were resigned. People accepted their place in life. They did not even try to make their children work hard in school; I can't remember any child being pressurised.

John   I suppose at that period you were glad to have any sort of job. A perfectly accepted excuse for not coming to school was, 'My boots – it was always "boots" -- are at the menders.' It was quite acceptable.

About the Centre school, Olive wrote:

> I have very little knowledge of other 'progressive' schools of the time; but the Centre school must have been different if only because the children were different. All the parents who sent their children to it were very involved members; most of the children would have attended the nurseries. Being a child in the Centre was being part of an extended family.

John wrote:

> My early and continuing personality development was enormously influenced for the good through my family membership of the Centre. The results obtained in terms of personality development and improved 'health' were absolutely astounding.

[John and Olive visit old Centre friends when they come back here on holiday.]

Pam and Harold (Adge) Elven [Their families were members for three or four years before the outbreak of war and rejoined afterwards, when Adge joined the staff part-time. He worked on the 'social floor' three or four evenings a week. In order to start work at the Centre at 4.30pm he took the opportunity to work 'staggered hours' in his Civil Service job, beginning every morning at 8am. He was, when he retired, a Higher Executive Officer in the Ministry of Education. Pam was a secretary. Adge's father was a porter with Road Carriers.]

Adge   I'd take over from Olive Fee, or we would work together, giving out tickets to the children and getting them back, and afterwards, when the children had gone, recording what was on them. I had to show new members round, and listen to the others and forward their ideas to Mary or Amy. I'd say, 'It must come from you, we're not starting anything, but if enough of you are keen, space will be made available.' This was Doc's philosophy. Because the parents asked, I ran a swimming class.

Pam   I remember, you didn't believe in teaching them till they had got full confidence in the water itself. He would come out and he would be red and scratched all over where the children had climbed all over him – you couldn't see him for children. He would throw them and toss them.

Adge   Yes, we used to go into the shallow end of the big pool and we used to romp. I did this for several weeks and then one day I said, 'Now we are going to be serious.' And they quickly learned to swim.

When the children came from school, one of us would station ourselves down between the gym and the learners' pool and another out on the outside play area.

Pam The closing was a tragedy. It closed a month before we were married. We never knew it as a married couple – something I had always dreamed of. I longed to have children and to bring them up in the environment of the Centre. It was something that was very important to me. I used to walk past the dreadful shell of a building and feel very sad that I was no longer part of it.

When my family joined, I was about eight and my sister was little. I loved to take her to the nursery and see the babies. It was a children's paradise. But I was always a bit of a loner. I used to go to the Centre most afternoons and I enjoyed using things I never had of my own like bicycles and roller skates. I was not allowed to go in the water much because I had ear trouble. When we rejoined after the war, I did not come to the Centre much for quite a time, but after I got to know Adge and he taught me to swim and play badminton, I changed and became quite sociable.

Adge I was 12 when we joined. I had to nag and nag my parents to go along and see the place. They joined for my sake. They never used it very much. My father worked terribly long hours. I was often in bed and asleep before he came home. And my mother did not like going on her own. [Later Adge remembered that his mother learned to swim.]

You could see every activity that was going on. I'd never seen a gym used in the way the one in the Centre was. You could watch the people playing badminton from the viewing window. A group of us children started playing badminton. We used to play from 6 till 7 or 7.30. Then when the seniors chased us out we went into the gym, just leaping about, swinging on the ropes and devising our own games. We used to spend quite a lot of time moving all the apparatus exactly to our liking before playing 'Off Ground'.

Another thing I remember, we used to stand on the vaulting box and dive, and grab the stationary rope and swing. When we had all had a turn, we would move the box back six inches and try again and go on till we had all dropped out. I remember one chap Eric Booth who missed the rope and fell flat on the floor – and he bounced! (it was a sprung floor). When he got his breath back, he carried on. We used the apparatus generally as it should not be used. We just played. Then, at the 8 o'clock bell we ran up the stairs to the swimming pool and had our half hour's swim. After that we got a snack or a drink of lemon at the cafeteria and tucked ourselves into a corner of the Long Room for a little, and then went home. Sometimes we played a little table tennis or snooker, and of course there was dancing. A chap called Pettifer, he started a dancing class for the juniors. I learned all the dances when I was 14. He taught us all the main steps and then variations. After the war, I ran classes for the youngsters in my turn.

It was the sheer informality of the whole thing that attracted me. Within reason we could do what we liked, and that was the attraction. These physical activities let out all the built-up frustrations from school. My homework suffered and I struggled later, but you could do homework there; there was the 'library' upstairs where you could sit and write. Homes didn't always have a quiet place. It was all there, a whole wide spectrum.

It was a great place for mixing people who met and socialised. The cross section was fantastic – dustmen to lawyers. People of natural interests used to gather together. We had clubs within the club.

Although I was on the staff, I was very much a member, ready to get involved in anything. I was friendly with my father-in-law before the war. After the war he used to play piano and I'd do MCing for dances.

Pam   One of the Mulvaney twins played the piano too and the other was on drums. There was John Smith on the cornet and we had a bass player and others.

I think we were a healthy lot of children. The babies all seemed to be so beautiful. ... The children did not have much respect for the equipment.

Adge   Doc did not want them to have respect for the equipment. He did not like them breaking things deliberately, but he was interested in seeing what they would do with the equipment.

Pam   I think nowadays people would be prepared to pay quite a sum of money just to know where their children are.

Adge   There was a hooligan element that forced themselves in. But there was none of that among the members. We had to go to the rescue of the gatekeeper quite often – he was old; he had a marvellous memory and knew nearly everybody. When he did not know them, he asked to see their membership cards, but sometimes people just barged through and I would have to go to his assistance. I was quite husky in those days, and I could call on any of the rest of the lads.

Pam   When it closed, the Centre was just getting established as far as the outside world was concerned. There was a series of television programmes right at the end. Various interviewers came down. Wynford Vaughan Thomas was one, I think. John Ellison interviewed Adge and me, and my parents were interviewed, and several other families.

Adge   I noticed the children seemed to set themselves goals. For instance one would dive and dive every day, getting more skilled and then suddenly give it up for a while and spend his time on something else, and then come back to it.

     The children had freedom to choose. It was interesting to see the pattern of activity of the children – when they joined, rushing about and trying everything and then settling into an individual pattern. They were all searching all the time for what they wanted. I am sure this was Scott Williamson's intention. He was super, I loved him almost like a father; not that I want to put my own father down. I thought a very great deal of him. I was in awe of him at first, then, after the war, I realised what a great man he was. The staff used to have meals together and I used to listen to wonderful conversations about the concept of the Pioneer Health Centre and what he was aiming for. Strong arguments used to go back and forth between him and Innes Pearse. Lots of it was above my head. I really looked up to both of them. They were true professionals. He could listen too. He would say, 'Come on boy, lets walk round.' And he would ask me questions about what we saw and about people he did not know and then listen to me – to my opinions. He never talked down to you. In the canteen, wholemeal bread was there and at table, when we were talking, he would say, 'I believe this is better.' He wouldn't lay down any strictures, he'd pass an opinion.

Pam   We saw our Centre friends often after it closed in 1950; not so much after we had children. When we moved out of Peckham in 1956 we lost touch with them.

In a letter, Pam wrote:

My present feelings about the Centre are two-fold. I am proud to have been part of the Peckham experiment, also sad because the experiment was cut short. Not only was it a loss to science, but the unique opportunity to go forward as a parent in the experiment was lost to me personally.

There was most certainly a feeling of belonging to a community, and close relationships were formed with joys and sorrows shared.

Mr Charles Stockwell [Pam Elven's father, aged 80 at the time of the interview. An undertaker with his own business.]

Our family were some of the original 'guinea pigs'. I soon found my fondness for games – billiards, table tennis, badminton – and amateur dramatics. Without the Centre, I doubt if I would have taken up these recreations. Fishing was more or less my favourite hobby.

The Centre offered opportunities for latent talent. When I used to play snooker, there was a young girl of about twelve years old used to watch. She was almost leaning on the table one day and I asked her if she would like a game. She said, 'I'd love one.' I could see she had talent. We gave her the opportunity to play and she developed, and later was a well-known snooker player. Her name was Maureen Barrett. That is one illustration of the opportunities the Centre offered. I found, with myself, playing all the games and improving my skill, I enjoyed playing so much more. This applied too to the amateur dramatics; I discovered I had a flair for acting. Swimming did not appeal to me. I only entered the pool once. After the war, I used to play the piano for dancing. I composed a waltz. I used to play it on Saturday nights – a special waltz for the Centre. The biggest thrill in my life was when I went to see the Centre film and it opened up with my tune played by a full symphony orchestra. There it was – my tune, my waltz; someone got it orchestrated. My hair stood on end with the thrill. The film was not really very good; it didn't really show what life was like at the Centre.

One thing my wife and I were both grateful for was the periodic health overhaul.

I am certain there was a feeling among the members of being proud to belong to the Centre, and there was a great love of the two doctors who, to my mind, were very exceptional characters.

If there was one wish I could be given, it would be to go back in time for a year at the Centre in either period. They were extremely happy years.

Mr and Mrs Loughlan

The children brought us in. It was a beautiful place. Children had a lovely time there.

We could mix with other families. Children said, 'This is my Mum, this is my Dad.' There were families round about with children of the same age. They used to call for one another and go off together.

Mr and Mrs Foard [Joined before the war]

Mrs F   Relations belonged and when they extended the area we joined. Most of the whole family belonged to it. My husband earned £2:9s then. We paid one shilling a week to belong; but it was worth it. It was lovely because most of our relations came from this area. We could all meet Saturday night or one night a week instead of having to go around to each other's houses. Some relations had children of school age who used to go there from school and have tea – used to have a bun or something.

I had a boy of 18 months when we joined. I used to put him in the nursery (we paid twopence and they were given tea with milk from the farm and spinach) about twice a week, and go to Keep Fit and then swim.

The check-up was wonderful. There were four doctors, two ladies and two gentlemen. The whole family got a check-up. The doctors seemed to be more interested in you than doctors are usually. You could ask them if you were worried about the children at all.

Mr F   You knew the children were all right. You didn't worry about them. You could go round there and the children could go there. You might not see them but you knew they were all right.

Mrs F   [Main benefits] Meeting friends and relations, and it got you out of the house. And the nursery, so you were free for a couple of hours – the children not under your feet. It was good for them too to be away from you.

It was quite a trot from here, but it was all right with the baby in the pram, and we were young then, we didn't mind walking.

Saturday nights we danced up there, and on Monday
nights we used to go to learn to dance. I thought it was a
marvellous place.

It would be lovely to have one in each area. You would
be able to get to know the neighbours and the little children.
It would unite people.

Mr F   There was no getting bored. All the family found something
to do.

Gladys and Elvet Chapman [Elvet was a boy (aged 10 to 15) before
the war. His father walked from South Wales to London during the
Depression, to find work. He got a job as an oxyacetylene welder,
found a flat in Peckham and fetched his wife and son. Elvet was a
footwear sales assistant. Later he was a custodian at the Houses of
Parliament.]

Gladys   We had many a good Saturday night up there.

Elvet   There were always new things to do at the Centre, like the
trampoline in the grounds.

If we were running around after 8 o'clock up and
down the stairs we were stopped and asked who we were
with. If it was our mother or father we were told to go
back to them. So after that we tried to attach ourselves to
an adult.

Before the war came (when I was 15) we started to learn
to dance, slow foxtrots, tangoes, English waltz etc. I learned
to swim in the learners' pool and became mad on diving.
[Towards the end of the war, when he was stationed in
Austria, he represented his battalion in high diving competitions.] I remember there was a turnstile – a green one –
between the toilets and the changing room. You got a shiny,
silver-coloured, penny-sized disc from the Cash Desk in
exchange for your 'ticket'.

My Dad was a darts enthusiast; he ran the Darts Club.

Dr Williamson was so warm and friendly. Used to
mooch around the building, put his hand on your head and
say, 'Getting on all right?' You had a different sort of
relationship with him than you had with a doctor usually,
when you felt like a 'case' – not a person, not friendly.

Mrs Olga Reade [née Smith, was a schoolteacher and finished her
career as head of the Infants department of a large Primary school. She
married just after the Centre closed.] She wrote:

The Smith family joined when the area was extended to include the other side of the main road. For my parents, it was the unique opportunity of the annual health overhaul that made it attractive.

As a teenager, it was the comradeship that the physical activities such as badminton, swimming, gymnastics and dancing engendered. My mother encouraged me to go only after my homework, piano and violin practices were completed.

Our home was bombed, but after the war we returned to Peckham to my grandfather's house, and rejoined the Centre. By then I was teaching in Greenwich. I was very lucky to be chosen to play a leading part in the Centre film. That was a marvellous experience.

My understanding of the importance of the family led me to help to start a 'Family Club' which we began at Rangefield School on the Downham estate in the late 1970s. This use of the school one evening a week where the whole family could come and enjoy various activities or just meet and talk was recognised by the then Education Officer, Dr Briault, for the ILEA.

To put it in a nutshell, the Centre enriched our lives – for good.

Mrs Lily Mears and Mrs May Burnett [Mr Mears was an electrician and Mr Burnett had his own barber's business. Both families moved to the country (Somerset) a few years after the closure of the Centre.] Lil said she had asked her son what he could remember:

Lil   He was four and a half when the Centre finally closed. 'It was lovely because we never wore any shoes – and you used to let me do it at home.' And he remembers the little pool and learning to dog paddle.

May   The Doctors were lovely; they were so feeling; they were not like doctors or scientists; they were one of you. It was so lovely on a Saturday evening. You used to go up and, if you wanted to, you could dance or swim or, if you wanted a cup of coffee, you could sit by the side of the pool. My husband worked till 8 o'clock weekdays so we could only go together on Saturday evenings; we used to bring Michael; he was eight or nine.

Lil   All the things that brushed off on us at the Centre – from the way Dr Pearse handled the babies and the nurse handled them too. When we moved down here, country life took the place of the Centre; I joined the Women's Institute, the local Methodist chapel, ran bazaars and fund-raising efforts, helped to run a kindergarten in the village hall – it was all voluntary; it was going back to the Centre without knowing it, living as a group.

For some years I ran a Children's Home. I would not

have had the courage or the wisdom for that if I had not been at the Centre. When I took the children to the dentist, he said, 'I have much less to do for your children's teeth.' He said, 'I wonder why this is?' I didn't try to explain about the Centre but I had picked up some knowledge about diet there, plus courage. You got a sense of being your own self. You got the habit of thinking, 'I could do that.' You got the power to take responsibility. I am sure I have done much more with my life.

It taught us to let go. I can remember when I first saw Michael climbing up the side of the gym and Doc Willy came along and told me to stand back from the window: 'You are communicating your fears to him; in fact, you should go away or you may make him fall.' My instinct was to dash down there and fetch him down. Doc said, 'He knows what he is doing; he is perfectly capable of doing it, or he would not attempt it; but he'll only get down again if you go away.' I remember when Michael went to the Centre school, and he wanted to go to the corner of the road – where the van picked him up – on his own. I used to stand in my porch and watch, and he used to turn round to see if I was still there and gesture to me to go back in. That was what the Centre was all about; it taught us to let go.

It was very sad when the Centre had to close. I remember endless meetings. So many people tried and fought so hard. We just couldn't believe that people could be so stupid as to let a place like that fall apart. There again, I think it has left its mark, if people are still talking about it 30 or 40 years afterwards. It made you sort out your talents that are dormant in all of us. It wasn't built for our benefit. Nevertheless it provided opportunities for us all; it was there to use; no-one made you do anything, but if you saw something and it suddenly stirred you to some kind of action...

May

Lil

Yes it was sad when the Centre closed – very sad. We had moved from north London so that we could belong to the Centre.

My son remembers the babies' swimming pool. It was emptied every day and the water started running in at 2 o'clock when the Centre opened. We used to stand and watch and my Mike used to sit in it in a few inches of water and he used to turn over with his hands on the

May

bottom and walk along on his hands and float with his face in the water, but he used to quickly put his face up and breathe. He was doing dog paddle at six months.

May   I really enjoyed just sitting down in the Cafeteria and just having a chat to anyone who came by. I used to do Keep Fit and play a bit of badminton. I must be honest and say I never succeeded in learning to swim, though I tried.

If you belonged to the Centre, you always had lots of friends. In London you can live without knowing your neighbours, and as for the people on the other side of the road, you'd never know them. In the country, its different; you know everybody and you ask the people you meet in for a cup of tea. When we lived in Peckham, you hardly spoke half a dozen words. Everybody was in a hurry.

Lil   We used to use the night nursery sometimes after Dr Pearse said that babies usually sleep just as well in their prams as in their cots at night. But my husband was often away on a job during the week. It was Oakley that was the Centre for him. We went camping there every summer – nearly every weekend from Easter to October – and often Michael and I used to stay there during the week as well.

The camping continued after the Centre closed, when Mary Langman was running the farm.

We used to weed the kitchen garden and help Mary out with picking the fruit when she had to get some to the market in Bromley. The men built some new pigsties for Mary and if she wanted any jobs done, lots of us were do-it-yourself people. My Walt would offer to do the electrics and Wally Arnold was a bricklayer and others helped. We had great fun. In those days in the building trade a foreman was called a coddy. Wally Arnold was a coddy. We used to brew up for them and we used to call, 'Tea up. All stop.' And they said, 'We can't stop; we are in the middle of a mix.' Wally Arnold said, 'This has gone on long enough; in my trade only the foreman decides when to stop for tea. He wears a bowler hat and he has a whistle and we stop for tea when he takes off his bowler hat and blows his whistle.' So next weekend someone produced a bowler hat and I brought a whistle. It used to be a marvellous sight. They all used to wear just a pair of trunks or old khaki shorts. And when they started to work, Wally Arnold said, 'Where's me bowler?'

and he'd say, 'We are not going to stop for tea till I raise my bowler and blow my whistle.'

My Michael asked one day, 'Where do babies come from?' He was only four or five. I said, I am going to ask Alec if he has got a pig that is about to farrow. If you can watch, you will know how babies are born. I asked Alec and he said, 'I have got one sow who is not very temperamental. But supposing it is in the middle of the night?' I said, 'It doesn't matter; wake us up.' In fact it was at 4am. It was light, it was summer. She had thirteen babies and it was wonderful to watch them crawling round on to the teat. My Michael's face was a picture. And that satisfied him for a long time until he wanted to know how the seeds got there in the first place.

In the summer after we moved here, Michael said, 'I don't like it here as much as I used to. I can't go camping here.' So we put the tent up at the bottom of our bit of orchard. We had an Alsatian pup by then. And Michael used to come home from school, collect his rations and the two of them used to disappear into the orchard. He wouldn't sleep indoors at all in the summer.

We had great fun at Oakley. Michael and I used to stay the whole summer holidays. We always used to take care of the field. We never left our tents up in the same place for more than a couple of nights, so as not to spoil the pasture. We took it in turns to clean the loos and the two showers we used.

There was one interesting thing. There were never any flirtations or scandal. Of all the years we went – 20 odd families, there was never a row about anyone looking twice at anyone else's wife or husband. No popping in behind the bushes.

May   My Michael used to go to Oakley on his own sometimes. He had his own tent.

May Rossiter [Joined in 1946 with her van-driver husband and two small children]

It was a happy place. I can't think of anybody being really grumbly. I used to go there for the whole afternoon and really enjoyed it. Gladys Coring's children I used to know very well and the Bishops. You got friendly with people who had children of the same age.

The Centre was a big thing for me. I used to swim a lot

– when I was expecting our fourth child too. I got a certificate for swimming a quarter of a mile...

The doctors helped me a lot. They were wonderful when there was something wrong with any of the children. You didn't mind going and telling them anything, did you? You didn't feel they were a cut above you. They would tell you the truth; doctors used not to always in those days...

I had three children then, and one day I felt terrible. I couldn't even wash a nappy. Bruce was under a year. I felt, 'Hurry up and open Centre and I'll be down there.' I took the children to the nursery and Mrs Collins looked at me. She said, 'You need to see the Doctor,' and I said, 'I'm all right.' She said, 'Well, you sit there.' Later she said, 'The doctor's free now.' They said, 'You have got appendicitis. You'll have to go into hospital.' I said, 'I can't go. What about the children?' And they said, 'What is the Centre for? They'll be all right.' The children were looked after. The woman who was helping in the nursery, she had Stella. Mrs Collins, being a nurse, took Brian, and Mrs Patterson had the baby. She lived in the same street, so my husband had the baby at night and took him along in the morning.

My children liked going without their shoes. In the summer they used to run across to the Centre from here with just their little shorts on.

What was good about the Centre was that we had no bath – and we still have no bath – but then we could go over and have a bath straight from here; you collected the cleaning things so you could clean it after.

There were great days at the farm with the children. They used to watch the cows. We didn't camp. We used to go for the day.

You had to join as a family. I think that is good because it brings the husband in. I go to a church and my husband does not go, but he used to go to the Centre.

Stella and Brian went to the Centre school. It was a very good school for Brian because he was slow. He was a plodder. When he went to Hollydale School he never finished anything, because he was slow. He still is, but he gets it correct in the end. He is well up in work now. He is a site manager for a builder. A freedom school was very good for him.

It didn't worry me that the doctors were studying you. After all, that's what they were there for, weren't they?

They were fathoming human beings – getting to the depths of them.

The Centre was a place that all the family liked to go to. That was the main advantage.

Mrs Ethelyn Hazell [From a letter she wrote to me last year. She joined with her policeman husband in 1935 just before the birth of her son.]

> The overhauls were more than welcomed by my family and it had the effect of alleviating any imaginary fears one might have had, and certainly I became a much fitter person as the years passed from my association with the Centre. I think the relief of being examined and knowing there was nothing fundamentally wrong was great. I can remember coming out of our first family consultation and the feeling of relief and elation.
>
> I am aware that, in a number of cases, the idea of an annual overhaul when you were not ill was frightening. I know some people resigned because they did not wish to be examined.
>
> My understanding of the whole real side of the work of the Pioneer Health Centre began when I was called to go and help Miss Langman with some typing when the Doctors were working on *Biologists in Search of Material.* They had seen me typing downstairs in the Cafeteria for a sketch we were doing in the Concert Party. I was very interested, and my whole attitude towards bodies, mothers, babies etc underwent profound change – for the better of course. I always wish I could have had a second baby during my time at the Centre, as my whole attitude had been changed through their teaching and influence. I thought it was all quite marvellous. Having once started typing some of their work, I was, and have been for the rest of my life, 'sold' on it.

[Ethelyn was one of the young mothers who lived with their children at Oakley House during the first year of the war (see her account in Chapter 4). For the rest of the war she was in the Land Army. Her husband was killed in 1943, and in 1947 she bought a 64-acre farm with a Land Army colleague in a steeply hilly part of Devonshire. They farmed entirely organically and very successfully for 16 years, building up a dairy herd, breeding race horses, keeping pigs and chickens and growing all the food for the amimals and themselves. Ethelyn later wrote a monograph in which she described her experiences.*]

John and Margaret Nash [John was a commercial artist. Margaret's father was Export Manager with Raphael Tuck.]

Margaret wrote:

> The health Centre days were a very long time ago. I was eleven when it opened. We were always keen to rush to the Centre after school, picking up our swimming things on the way. Firstly, we had a session in the gym

* *Running a Farm the Organic Way*

with Miss Crighton. This I enjoyed, but not so much when they were later abandoned and people did their own thing. I learned to swim in the 'small' bath with Mrs Shingles, but I must have been pretty confident because, at the end of my first lesson, she took me straight up to the 'big' bath where I swam a width straight away. Afterwards we would spend our few coppers in the cafeteria. I remember the lovely 'Scofa' bread at a penny a slice and the delicious lemon barley water also only one penny a beaker.

I can remember my mother being very proud of the fact that she learned to swim at 46. Special permission was given for the Centre to be opened early on Sunday morning for the keen swimmers to have a dip. The Moody boys [sons of a local GP] were all keen on this, and I believe they had the key to open up. I mean early – we went as a family at 6.30 and then my parents would often go on to church for eight o'clock communion. We used to go to the Moodys' house at 6am and wake them up.

John and I met at the camp at Sissinghurst, but I was only 14, and then the war came. We married a year after the war finished. We spent more time then making a home than attending the Centre, although John did scene painting for the Drama group and we both swam quite a lot and went dancing. Once I became pregnant, the Centre came into its own. We had had a pre-marital consultation with the doctors and then a pre-natal one. Dr Pearse sent me to Mrs Collins for advice on baby clothes. She supplied us with the Dayella to get cracking with making nighties and smocked dresses for the new infant. This was not my strong point, so I took my mother along to Mrs Collins' classes hoping to shelve some of this job – but in the end, I did do it all myself and mother did dressmaking for *her*self. We had such happy evenings up in the 'Nursery' and Mrs Collins was so very helpful. Unfortunately, the Centre closed when our son, Peter, was only a year old. But during that year I made a number of friends and am still in touch with quite a few of them to this day.

Now that I have grand-children and hear mention of their visits to the clinic or the doctor, or that they have to go out because the lively youngsters get bored at home, I do so wish they had the opportunity of using 'the Centre' and all the facilities that went with it. I know there are these leisure centres around and our son has one quite near, but as far as I can gather it is only for swimming they use it. It was the medical side of the 'Centre' that was such a boon to its members. We were indeed very fortunate.

John wrote:

The Centre spirit of the pre-war period was no myth. It was very real. I for one have much cause to be thankful for it. I sometimes feel that this spirit has run like a golden thread through our marriage.

Ann and Will Watson, Lilly and Ted Kelsey and Rose Runacres [They were all members pre-war and rejoined post-war. Mr Watson was a shipwright and later a director of a firm operating pleasure steamers on the Thames. Ted Kelsey was a salesman for a surgical instrument maker; Mrs Runacres' husband was a courier, mostly in this country, for a shipping line.]

Lilly	I think the most wonderful thing was that we all joined as a family.
Ann	Well, Will joined but he never came to any of the things there. He had to come to have an examination but he didn't join anything.
Ted	It was so nice to be able to go there and be able to meet each other; and also you could have a little meal, you know, a help-yourself meal, and then you could sit round and have a chat and if you didn't want to do that you could go and have a swim or anything else that was going on.
Lilly	You could talk to the doctors, couldn't you? They were friends.
Ann	It was one on its own. I don't think you can ever get one like it. We never had a lot of money in those days. We had £2.10s a week. I hadn't a penny to bless myself with on a Thursday. We walked everywhere; we had no money for the bus. We could go to the Centre for a few coppers a week. If we played badminton, it only cost us about threepence and then we could go upstairs and have a cup of tea for a penny, and sit; we looked forward to it so much. Then, afterwards, if you had time you could go and have a swim for another twopence, or threepence for a bath. John would have his tea in the nursery and I would take him home and it would be time for his bath and bed. He had been happy and was quite tired by then and I had been happy – I was contented, it made us all contented. In the evenings, mothers and fathers could leave their baby in the nursery and then they could dance or play badminton or anything, together.
I went back after the war. John was a schoolboy then, about ten, but he couldn't enjoy it so much because we were further away; he couldn't go straight from school, and he had homework.
The Radfords got married after meeting each other there; lots of them did.
Lilly	It was run by the people. Every activity was run by somebody that joined the Centre. My husband ran the badminton. But some people took advantage – I did see people on

nights when we had parties, where they passed drinks over their heads and never troubled to pay.

Rose   I do feel that we did want a bit more discipline. Especially the children.

Ann   It was lovely to see the little ones in the swimming pool; they had a children's swimming pool, and adults could go down there too; if you had never swum and you were afraid to go in the big pool you could always go down to the little one.

Lilly   There were three lovely doctors, they were scientists really. Really and truly we never appreciated it enough while we had it. Now you look back and think how lucky we were and the friendships we had. Of course, there wasn't only the sports side, there was quite an educational side as well.

Rose   It was always sort of health foods we had there; lovely little salads they would make summer or winter. And our bread was cooked there. We never had cups, we had bowls, and we had a little tray with a hollow in it for the bowl and the other part was our plate so everything could be sterilised. They had great big machines at the back of the kitchen.

Well, I think that the good thing that came out of all this is that all those years from the wartime we are still good friends, we all kept in touch with each other all these years. I didn't have any friends before. I wasn't a good mixer at all. I was terrible really, that's why, when I first joined the Centre, I left again – because I couldn't talk to people, but once I got in with the badminton and my husband began playing darts. With children, you got talking with mothers, and gradually I got into it. Once you get into a little group you can't just sit back can you? You have got to have a little bit of a say, and it really brought me out.

I don't think the girls remember it all that well. I think they remember the swimming more than anything, and the gymnasium; they used to like to be in the gym.

I remember, Mrs Brunker learned to swim after she was 60 and she used to jump off the top board. Doc Willy used to say, 'I wish she would hold her nose.'

Queen Mary came. She used to love to see the babies, and we had a window at the top of the badminton and they could look at us playing. The Duke of Kent came once too. We all turned out in our white. He seemed rather shy and said, 'Do you all come on the same afternoon?'

To make children and everybody appreciate things, you must pay a certain amount in, because anything that's free nobody appreciates do they?

Mrs Grier [Her husband was in the police force.]

The doctors and the members got on extremely well. There was no question of doctor and patient at all. One sort of always is in awe of doctors but certainly not with them. They were most friendly, at least we always found them so. They knew too where to send you if you had something that needed treatment. Dr Pearse arranged for me to go to the Elizabeth Garret Anderson.

I think it was a marvellous thing for families. It gave Colin a freedom he wouldn't have had. We used to let him go down there alone whereas we wouldn't have let him go elsewhere.

We are still friends with people we knew there.

I used to go to badminton more than you did. I think it may have been because you ran the club at the church hall. Anyhow, shift work bars you from social life quite a bit really.

We had a lot of visitors, a lot of well-known people, some from abroad. General Smuts was one. But the good thing was that there was never any preparation made for them; they just came and saw it as it was, with the members doing the things they would normally do.

Wally and Bunny Arnold [Wally was a bricklayer – later a site manager for a builder.]

Bunny   The open plan nature of the building was a great thing. I do feel that that made quite a lot of difference to my life. Being an only child – my father died when I was little and my mother had to earn a living by sewing – I had little opportunity to meet people. You could join in with a group; you could just be one of them without really knowing them, and then you did get to know them. You could look and see that so and so was swimming or playing badminton or roller skating and join in.

Wally   We met before the war. I wasn't a member at the time. I used to hang about outside waiting for a friend to sign me in, I was 17 – and I saw Bunny, in her school uniform, going in and I said to myself, 'She is the girl for me. I'd like to marry her.' We did our courting at the Centre and married during the war.

Bunny   I remember I got a bit annoyed when he was always around, and then I began to miss him when he wasn't.

After the war we joined as a family with our two year old. Tony went to the nursery but I think he learned to swim in the big bath with us.

Wally   I remember how he used to jump in from the side and I used to catch him. He loved being with adults – young adults; we were the first of our friends to have a child. We had lots of friends – a tremendous group of friends. You had a group of friends from badminton and another from table tennis. You didn't drop one lot, you kept them although you had another lot. There were large groups and they would intermingle or not intermingle. I used to play the piano and when I showed up in the Long Room, people would say, 'Here's Wally; now we can have some dancing.' I didn't mind; I liked any chance to play.

Bunny   Then there was the camping lot. I think because we shared our lives so much on holidays and weekends, we were closer to them than to anybody. We have kept up with the camping crowd longer. We still keep in touch – send Christmas cards.

Wally   I think there is one word that describes it – happiness. Weren't they golden years, eh, when you look back? God... But you couldn't describe it to anyone. You can't get anyone to understand what it was like. It is impossible.

Bunny   You can't describe the atmosphere there was, can you?

Could there be another Centre today?

Wally   It would have to be run as a family club. Otherwise it would be a glorified youth club, and you would have to have big men walking around seeing that everyone was behaving.

Bunny   It would depend on what area you had it in. After a time I think people would appreciate the advantages it had to offer. A family membership would be essential: then, if people wanted to join, you could be fairly sure that they would be reasonably responsible.

Wally   Perhaps if Mum and Dad were there they would control their children. The other aspect that was important – there were no spirits sold there. But would that satisfy the young adult today?

Bunny   We used to walk home with a crowd or with one or two others when we were teenagers at the Centre. I don't think that parents would worry if young people had somewhere like the 'Centre to go to.

[A year or two after the Centre closed, Wally and Bunny answered an advertisement for a bricklayer to join a group intending to build houses for themselves.]

Wally   By the end of a year we had 26 members, including five bricklayers, five carpenters, two electricians and two plasterers.

We agreed to put down £50 each and to work an average of 22 hours a week. This meant every weekend and two evenings (for four and a half years) and we all took one week of our two weeks holiday at the end of July, finishing with the August Bank Holiday, so we could put in 10 days work. We had no machinery at all except a cement mixer. We did everything – all the digging – by hand. While we were collecting enough members, we used to go at weekends to a 'bomb site' and practise digging; those who were experienced taught those who had never used a spade before.

We had a legal document drawn up that included the obligation to continue to work until the whole 26 houses were finished, except for the painting and decorating which was largely done by the wives after people had moved in. We were lucky that the Mayor of Lewisham at the time was an architect and wished us well; he provided all the plans and drawings free. The LCC gave us an interest-free loan, paying it in instalments as we progressed. We built two houses at a time.

[Wally was the site foreman for the whole four and a half years.]

The Arnolds and Ron and Sally Woodhouse [Ron was a senior clerical assistant. They joined post-war.]

Sally   We heard of the Centre from the people who were put in our house by the Council: our house in Brockley was requisitioned. They took four rooms from us before you could say knife. Later the Council commandeered another room; I still have it in for them for that. Doc Willy, bless his heart, tried hard to get that room back for us; he said there wasn't room for our two children in one bedroom.

It took us a long time to get down to the camp. As far as we were concerned, it wasn't us. Yet we loved it. I remember stooking [standing sheaves of corn on end to dry] and really enjoying it. The Centre brought out different bits of you. We all sort of grew and expanded in ways you would never have thought of. We did so many different things, even Ron, who didn't like making a fool of himself, he did everything except swimming. We were all part of it. When we first joined, I remember I was surprised that there were so many different types of people there, all getting on so well.

Bunny   I remember we used to get very worked up because the kids carved their initials on the tables. We thought it was like murder. But Doc Willy wouldn't step up the supervision. He said to one group of children – he never found out who was doing it – 'You're very silly children because these are your tables. They are not mine. They are yours.'

Sally   One of the things I remember there was the lovely atmosphere. Whereas you normally get some backbiting, I don't remember any – of course, you wouldn't be human if there were not some people you liked better than others – a lot of kindliness went on; a lot of help.

Bunny   The Centre was your life, wasn't it? I felt it was. My Mum used to say, 'I don't know why you don't take your bed down there.'

Sally   We had lots of parties. In our house in New Cross, we were always having parties of members and in other people's houses too. Once the whole of the swimming club turned up.

Gladys and Harry Coring [Joined soon after the war with boy of five and girl of eighteen months. Harry was a boiler maintenance man.]

From a letter from Gladys:

You use the word 'community'; the Centre needs a much warmer word than that; we did feel mutually responsible for each other. The Centre became an extension of our home – not a clinic or a leisure centre, nor was it political, racial or class motivated etc, but a place where the family could expand as a whole, and all in one building.

Some families first joined for the sports, others for the nursery facilities etc, but once inside that building there was a feeling of complete relaxation, that I have never found in any community centre since. There can never be another true Peckham Centre, as the core to that was the two doctors who pioneered it – but how marvellous it would be if there was a 'Centre' in each neighbourhood, what a lot of today's problems would be solved. The biggest thing – the thing they got right – is you start from the family. Its no good just having a community centre or a club with doctors at one end.

Gladys   We joined because I wanted somewhere to take the children out of the horrible [basement] flat, and a bit of social life; we had no neighbours because of the bombing, and I liked swimming. I couldn't afford the nursery down the road.

Then we found we had to see a doctor. I never dreamed anything was wrong. Dr Pearse said I had anaemia, I said, 'I know.' (I was pregnant and was taking lots of little green pills.) Dr Pearse gave me other kinds of iron, but it made no difference, my blood was not absorbing the iron.

In the end they gave me liv·r injections. Then I was away. I only had six and I can remember how different I felt after only two or three.

I used to swim every day. I was embarrassed about being so obviously pregnant. The first time, I went in as soon as the Centre opened at 2pm and there was no-one about. I look a big towel and hung it over the rail of the steps in the shallow end because you had to walk the length of the pool right close to the glass wall with the cafeteria tables on the other side to reach the steps leading down to the changing room. I had a lovely swim and when I wanted to come out I found people had begun to come into the cafeteria and the Long Room. I thought, how the devil am I going to get out of the water without them seeing me. I didn't realise that I must have looked even funnier in the water, floating and swimming on my back which I like to do. But I soon lost my self-consciousness and left that towel in the changing room. My costume was a two-piece made of ex-navy blue serge. In 1947 it was impossible to get a swimsuit to fit me: no stretch fabrics then. Mrs Collins, the dressmaker who was also head of the nurseries, helped me to make it – kind of loose bloomers that came right over my bulge, and we faced a bra of mine. I was enormous and it must have looked extraordinary, but it was comfortable.

I swam up to the day that Val was born. Later Richard Dimbleby and Rex Alston were doing broadcasts on Saturday afternoons from the Centre. Richard Dimbleby had just had a baby and he interviewed me. He asked, 'Did you swim for the exercise?' and I said, 'No, swimming is just the thing I enjoy; its so relaxing and its the one thing you can do when you are pregnant. You float so beautifully for a start. You have no weight.' I have never done eight lengths straight off since, but I did them the day before Val was born. That is something we could really do with now – somewhere to swim when you are pregnant, and not feel self-conscious. At the Centre you did not feel self-conscious. Its not like going to public baths. And first of all you have got to find somewhere to put the children or else you have got to take them with you as my daughter has to do. And that puts you half way to not going, to start with. Then you have to find a time when its not full of parties of school children which, in London, is most difficult.

Some of the nursery children could swim almost before they could walk. I took Val into the little pool when she was just on the point of crawling and I laid her on the top step in one inch of water. She loved her bath at home and she started splashing away. So I took her frequently and stayed with her. There was a student there watching the toddlers. And then one particular day – I can see her now – she slipped into the deep water (about one foot) and both her little arms and legs were going like a little dog paddle – she did about five strokes. I couldn't get over it. She was about eight months. Joy was two years older. She learned at about the same time.

Joy went into the big pool with me at two and a half. I took her down to the shallow end but she saw the boys jumping off the high boards. Before I could get out of the water she was climbing up the ladder. I could not stop her. I thought she would go right to the top; so I said, 'That's high enough now, jump from there.' She jumped and she was ages coming up; she was fighting for breath. When she could speak she said 'More, more,' I said, 'You must not do that any more. The doctor says you musn't. You are too young. When you are three you can jump off the high board.' Afterwards Doc Willy said to her, 'I saw you in the pool and you're not yet three. If you practice with Mummy down in the shallow end, then by the time you are three you will be able to go off the high board, won't you?' That more or less sunk in, but I had to keep my eyes open, and I could never get a swim myself. After she was three she used to go off the top board. I had to be there. She could only do dog paddle and she used to be struggling for breath when she came up.

If they are going to keep up their swimming, they have to go three or four times a week.

Harry   Oh yes, I used to love the Centre pool. We used to go on Saturday afternoon. That used to be our social day. We used to have the children with us on a Saturday. They played outside or we went swimming together and played table tennis. Alan was five when we joined. We used to stay till seven or eight o'clock. We let them stay up late on a Saturday. In the week, I used to call at the Centre on my way home from work at about five o'clock and walk home with Gladys and the children.

Gladys   I remember one day there was thick snow and Harry was working late. We had moved to a prefab outside the district. It was well over a mile, nearer two and uphill every inch of the way. They said it was all right if it was within walking distance. Well, there was no other way of getting there. That day I had to drag the push chair. I couldn't push it, and Alan was hanging on. He used to go to the Centre on his own from school. The day Val was born, I walked home from the Centre after swimming, put the children to bed; did some washing, then I had a bath and cleaned the bathroom. I was snug in bed when the waters broke. I was soaked. I woke Harry. We had planned that he would ride down to the phone box on his bike, but found it had a puncture. He was running full pelt down the hill when two policemen stepped out. They picked him up by his elbows and ran with him while he got his breath enough to say, 'Must get to the phone; wife's having a baby.' The baby was born less than an hour after I got to hospital.

Harry   Gladys was never happier than during that pregnancy.

Gladys   I never felt so fit before or since. I can remember how well I felt. With the other two, I was so tired.

Joy went to the Centre school. We wanted a school that continued the nurseries. We had to have lots of meetings to thrash out all sorts of things. The children came home for lunch and we took them again in the afternoon. Their brothers and sisters or mothers or fathers would be at the Centre too, of course, in the afternoons. There were no restrictions; no child was ever told to sit down or stand up, and yet there were never any explosions of noise.

I learned an awful lot about the Centre after it closed. I used to sit for hours talking to Dr Pearse about things I didn't really understand till 20 years after. We went to the talks the Doctors gave in the Long Room but I liked the private talks. You could say, 'I don't understand,' and Doc Willy would pause and example it. Although at the time we used to call ourselves his guinea pigs, we thought the idea was a kind of medical thing where you try to find out why ten people got measles in one place and only one in another – more like a research thing is today. And that is how outsiders often do look at the Centre. Now I understand better, but its still impossible to get it across to other people.

When we joined, Joy had a twisted foot. She was about 18 months and not walking. Her foot turned right in. I took her to Great Ormond Street. They said she must wear boots which would force her foot straight. They were so heavy that she would not even try to walk with them on and would get in a terrible state. She had had gastro-enteritis and digestive troubles as a baby and a kind of malnutrition. She was tiny. Dr Pearse said, 'She has a lazy muscle. This muscle has not developed properly.' Then at the family consultation, I said, 'I can't see how she is going to walk *ever*, because she won't try with these on.' Dr Pearse said, 'Well, leave them off. The only thing to do with these shoes is to throw them away.' She made as if to throw them out of the window. I said, 'Don't do that, I haven't paid for them yet.' I was paying for them by instalments, a shilling or two a week. I kept them for ages. I finished paying for them but never went back to Great Ormond Street.

'She ought not to wear any shoes. She needs to climb so as to use the muscle.' Later, Doctor Williamson said, 'Joy is going into the gymnasium with the other nursery children. What we want to coax her to do is to climb up those wall bars.' I thought he was mad. Then one day, I was in the needlework class (at the end of the Long Room by the viewing window into the gym) and he came up and said, 'Come and look at this. Stand well back, don't let her see you.' She was at the top of the wall bars, gripping the bars with her feet as well as her hands. She became so keen on climbing that it was a bit of a problem – she had no fear, but her foot straightened up. To this day, none of my children wear shoes in the house. For a long time Joy took off her shoes when she got into school in defiance of the teacher. In the Centre nurseries, none of the children wore shoes or socks.

The Centre gave you confidence. So many individuals

you could think of who changed and got confidence. All the family seemed to open up.

Harry   It was all the people you got to know, not only the doctors, that helped.

There was one thing we did in the evenings, once a week. We joined the choral society. We couldn't sing; we had awful voices, but we thought we wouldn't be heard in a crowd. We were taught by a chiropodist. He was Jewish and he took us round to Jewish clubs and hospitals to sing. I really enjoyed the singing. If we couldn't both leave the children we took it in turns.

Gladys   After the Centre closed, we carried on with the school, but it was only for the children up to five. A couple of mothers would take the children swimming in the public baths. Then there was Oakley House. The Doctors were still there and Mary Langman was there and we still went camping there at weekends and in the summer holidays. There were 30 or 40 families in the camping group. That was a little bit of the Centre still. And we got to know each other very well; it was like being a huge family.

The Centre was like an extension of your home. You grew out from being just Mum and Dad and three kids in your own little home.

We really appreciated the overhaul. You'd soon get rid of all worries. At the family consultation, I remember asking silly little questions.

Harry   Dr Williamson was very human – no officialdom. The children would go up to the Doctors and talk to them.

Gladys   Dr Pearse passed me in the Long Room one day and she said, 'You do look nice today, Mrs Coring.' – She was a friend.

When I joined, I was very anti-clinics. We were six children and my mother felt she knew better how to look after us than the general run of doctors. I suppose I got it from her. But at the Centre, you could see the results of the things the Doctors taught, and that made you trust them.

We learned a bit about food. I had always been more concerned to see that the family were full up than whether it was doing them good. Then the children began to like the Centre bread because they had it in the nursery, so we bought loaves from the Centre, but it cost nearly twice as much as ordinary bread.

There were so many original and good ideas there – the babies' cots put on the floor that they could see out of, and roll out of when they were ready. The cups had no handles to get broken. The tables were a sort of V shape. You could fit them together and make a long table or else you could get four or five people round one.

The staff didn't tell people off, but the members did sometimes. If you saw an unruly child say painting the wall or banging at a window, you might speak to him or you might go to the mother and tell her. If some lads were monopolising the diving boards or jumping in one after the other and making a terrible splash, the other swimmers might ask them to let other people have a turn or to let the younger children use the deep end too.

If you have a community Centre and it closes down, within two years it's all forgotten. But no-one who's been a member of the Peckham Centre has ever forgotten it. We still write to Peckham friends, but we have all moved away. When the Centre was open, you would not move far away and you'd put up with atrocious conditions.

First you have got to have the right kind of building. Then you have got to have the right environment. You would have to have sufficient people who are interested and wanting the thing.

Chapter 8

Mrs Purser's Experience

I was married in January 1935, and within a few weeks we received an invitation to visit the Centre. My husband and I had been very curious as to the use the rather strange building was to be put. One of our mutual interests was building construction, and design of furniture. We knew very little on either subject, although we both considered that, in the thirties, design in this direction was at its lowest – so we were immediately attracted to the Centre building and all it contained.

Empty, the building meant very little to strangers; filled with the young and old, it was vibrant with life, and I was eventually to see that every hour from two o'clock to ten, had its own light and quality. When it was dark, and the lights were on in the building, from the outside it was as if a huge ship was floating by.

How, I thought, could one be so lucky, to marry and then be invited to use this building, the lovely swimming pool and other facilities? I had at that time no knowledge of the Doctors or their work. I had rather dreaded married life, for in those days, one had no job after marrying, one resigned on marriage. It had also meant giving up a number of activities connected with my previous employment, and living in a new neighbourhood. I had thought to be bored and lonely.

We made our separate appointments for the overhauls, and then the family consultation. I remember very little of the first overhaul. I do know that the staff must have been more than carefully chosen, everyone was kind and friendly. What I am trying to say is that I was considerably astonished at the atmosphere in the Medical Deptartment, I could choose my appointment time, I could ask questions, there was no rush to get rid of me. I was in fact, a personality, not just a number or another patient; I was ME.

Now we come to the crunch – our family consultation. My husband's results were perfect, he was a thoroughly healthy man. But me – down the list went Dr Pearse – low blood count, lack of calcium etc, etc. It was obvious to me, that having been seriously ill when I was 21, now, at 25, I had been cured of the actual disease, but I had little or no health; 'devitalised' Dr Pearse called my condition. And so, after many more questions to the Doctors, it was agreed we should not start a family until I was at my peak. Until then I would be fitted with a contraceptive cap.

The Doctors explained that it was not their intention to treat disorder: on the other hand, their research would be affected, unless the mothers-to-be, (and indeed the fathers) were in good health when conception took place.

So for a year I attended the Medical Department, all the necessary things were fed to me. I watched my diet, made my own bread from stone ground flour, and, when possible, purchased food grown at the Centre farm. To our delight, our second family consultation was very different from the first, and the Doctors said, 'Go ahead and start a family.'

A few months went by with no signs of pregnancy, so again I was taken in hand, and eventually one lovely day, never to be forgotten, an examination confirmed my pregnancy – Dr Pearse and I actually danced round the examination bed, and we soon had Dr Williamson and Sister in to give their congratulations, I don't think anyone could have had a lovelier start to a pregnancy.

During pregnancy I flitted in and out of the babies' and toddlers' nursery, discussed clothes with the sister in charge, and was allowed to handle the babies and help with odd jobs. This was tremendous, as I came from a small family, and had had no babies or young children around me. So, when my baby was born, no difficulties or terrors. Over the years I have seen young mothers terrified of handling their babies, and panic setting in when something was wrong.

We were by now fully part of the Centre although, as newly-weds, much of our time was spent setting up our home. I swam every afternoon, until the seventh month, and then only one thing stopped me. I couldn't get into a swim suit, I had managed for some time with my husband's suit plus a top of my own making, but eventually gave up. Every pregnant woman should be enabled to swim, it is gorgeous. After all these years, I can remember one simply floated on air; the only laughable snag was getting on to one's feet, prior to departing from the water.

I also organised and ran a concert party; we had the greatest of fun, and it filled a gap in my life (prior to marriage I had been studying at the Guildhall School of Music, and doing a great deal of singing locally). Now I was able to use my talents, which was extremely satisfying.

Dr Pearse had suggested that as I was having a normal pregnancy, perhaps I would like to have the delivery at home. She made no secret of the fact that pregnancy was not an illness, and confinements should not therefore take place in hospital. Of course she was right, most of the mothers-to-be that I mingled with in the Centre were at their peak, as I was – they carried their babies with great pride – and, although I have forgotten many of the day-to-day incidents, standing out as a vivid memory are certain mothers who radiated fitness and joy. One would miss someone for about a fortnight, then that new mother would walk the length of 'the cafeteria' (as we called one of the long rooms) with her baby – and there would be a rush to see and exclaim on the new member.

Then I made a mistake I have bitterly regretted; having no sisters or relations around, I decided to go into hospital. So I went into Kings College Hospital in Denmark Hill. I was brimming with happiness and health. The baby would complete everything, I felt. I looked forward with confidence to the birth. Sad to say I hated every minute there, and had the most harrowing of confinements. I had difficulty in explaining what had happened, when talking to Dr Pearse, but after a number of very fit mothers also complained, we all realised our experience was no unusual thing.

After the birth of my son, I was soon around again. I was able to continue with the Concert Party because the Centre had a night nursery. There was a routine for this, baby was undressed and made ready for bed, but instead of the cot, was put into the pram, wheeled down the road and into the night nursery and left with Sister until we were ready to leave. My baby never knew he had been out of the house.

One of the first lessons I was to learn was through the Concert Party. My young friends of the party, mostly teenagers, became very interested in my baby, and very quietly admired. After all, they had been with me two evenings a week for nine months, supported me physically as well as mentally, they were part of him. I began to realise that for the successful growth of society all must come together, the young in years, the old, the girls, the fellows, the single, the married. Maybe on reflection, this was where I became completely involved and interested in the Experiment, so little I understood, so much I wanted to know. But at least I had, I thought, settled my future, I no longer aspired to a professional career as a singer, here was something far more important, of which I could be part.

In the afternoons my baby was taken into the nursery, while I met friends, and took part in various activities. By this time others were looking after nursery teas, and helping Sister with the feeding. I took my turn, and got to know all the babies. I watched their growth and development from new babies to toddlers. My own son enjoyed every moment in the nursery. By the time he was taking his first staggering steps, he knew the way from the pram park to the nursery, and was away with his bag containing 'spares', before I had finished parking the pram.

I became very adept at managing toddlers who were not yet using a spoon, although on solids. I could after much practice deal with six round a table, spooning each in turn, great fun, although we all had a dread of 'junket' days – terrible stuff to deal with!

There was a regular clinic for babies: feeding and weaning were discussed. Almost all of us breast fed our babies. Everything for me was easy, and Tony more or less weaned himself, and, by seven months, had completely naturally finished with the breast.

Clothing for the babies and toddlers was very much talked about, and I often found myself arguing with others who just couldn't bear the thought of leaving pretty petticoats etc off.

Dr Pearse also disliked 'sore bottoms'; she blamed the rubber pants and disliked them intensely. Fortunately I had seen some sore bottoms in the nursery before I had my own baby, so I never once used rubber pants. I had a lot more washing, some very dirty cot sheets, and some stained nightgowns, but always a beautiful baby's bottom, and incidentally a contented baby.

From what I have written, it would seem that it was I and not my husband using the Centre, therefore where was the family unit? The answer is in the newness of our family unit. My husband was studying hard, and also making furniture and fitments, while I helped with the painting. We were in fact very happy to be in our new home together, so apart from the concert party, we weren't to be seen there much in the evening, although, before our marriage, we had done a great deal of dancing. Such was the situation when the Centre closed at the outbreak of the war.

When the Centre reopened our family was at a different stage of development and we used the Centre very differently.

The following are notes about the post-war period:

When the Centre reopened, the members made their appointments for the overhaul. There was great excitement and pleasure, everyone looked forward to this. Our own family was no exception – Tony was 100 per cent, so was my husband – and I had managed to retain the standard I reached before and during pregnancy.

Tony settled into the Centre so easily: he followed the general pattern – concentrating on one skill until he himself was satisfied. Most of his time was spent in the gym or swimming pool. He had enough read- ing matter, paints etc, in our own home, so he mostly chose the activi-ties with movement and the companionship of other children. He would come each day from school which was a short distance away, and I was comfortably aware he was around, then home for supper and bed.

My husband was teaching at Evening School, so still didn't have much time, and whereas during the first phase we were busy making our home, now during the second life of the Centre, we were putting our home together again!

So when my husband went off in the evening to teach, Tony went to bed and I to the Centre; my husband finished his classes, called in home to see Tony was all right, and then joined friends and me in the Centre for a cup of tea, and then home together.

As you don't have to be told, the variety of families brought into the Centre many skills and expertise. We could always rustle up a dance band, and I can't remember a Saturday night without a dance in the long room.

Various groups put on plays, and very good they were, and well patronised by members. I produced and acted in quite a number, and from among the members we could find someone to make scenery, set up lighting etc, and men like my husband would be called in to any section and anywhere to do a particular skilled job.

Badminton was very popular both at afternoon and evening sessions, and players emerged good enough for County standard.

I was very much drawn to the upstairs games room, where there were billiards and darts – mostly when taking visitors round (the open plan you see worked!) I became fascinated with snooker, and after practice on the children's table was allowed by the members to play on the full-size table. From the day the Centre closed I have never played another game of snooker; there has been no opportunity.

There were matches arranged with other clubs by members in all our different sections. Darts were very popular, there was a ladies' section – I enjoyed very much playing against other clubs and entertaining them afterwards.

Table tennis also produced many good players. The following might interest. Always playing table tennis was a youngish man about 30 years old. He was not married, and obviously his family did not use the Centre much. He was a very good player and I soon tackled him about a bit of coaching. He was a hard taskmaster, but soon had me playing a reasonable game, so with his skill he was soon noticed by other members and in great demand. The young man didn't have much going for him in the way of looks and conversation, but he gained confidence, and was soon coming to the Saturday night dances. He turned out to be a very good dancer and he never lacked for partners.

'Adge' Elvin was a part-time staff member – apart from the youngsters who always wanted him to swim with them, he had continual dancing classes, and I became one of his willing 'stooges'. By that I mean a young fellow would be taught steps, and then practise with me, until he overcame his shyness and danced with one of the girls. I remember one young man who made a very slow start, and murdered my feet, but eventually became very good, and I would have to be quite humble and say, 'Don't I get a dance this evening?'

Saturday evening was the highlight of the week for me. The Long Room was so very right. The pillars hid the shy, the tables were matey – to have a beer or cup of tea and a good natter. I learned a great deal about people during these sessions. My husband was also a very good dancer, and I was lucky if I had a dance with him. I didn't mind in the least; it gave me time to circulate, talk and get to know the members.

We also had another hall on the upper floor, or we could use the theatre for mid-week dances. The various sections would run a dance during the week – for which we paid. We were a joyous crowd always ready for some celebration – which by the way didn't happen unless the members suggested and organised. For instance, there was always a St Valentine's dance – with appropriate decoration. It was so easy to arrange, because there was always a band available, always an MC and someone to arrange a programme and decorate the hall.

The children had a lovely party at Christmas, and the adults celebrated with a New Year party. A temporary committee would form and a theme emerge – the Cafe and Long Room being decorated accordingly. In the afternoons, for weeks before the New Year, we would make paper flowers etc, and the Centre building would be transformed. We also ventured into fancy dress costumes.

The Cafeteria staff were quite angelic with all the extra work involved, for of course we invaded the kitchen, being always self catering.

Mustn't forget water polo – once a week there was a match during the season, and if one was tardy it was hard to get a view of the play – very popular.

Whist drives of course, not my cup of tea!

And typing the above, I have just remembered – the children roaming around the Centre had come across a member of the staff holding a class for crafts. We thought the girls might be interested but the boys were too – my son presented me with a small leather purse with my initials stamped on it. It was a surprise. I had seen him interested, but had left well alone, and that was the result.

When I was answering visitors' questions, it was nearly always pointed out that it was mostly physical activity – from Church groups, why hadn't we a chapel? Why didn't we have Church services? The answer was of course that we as members could have had all that, if we had wanted – the Doctors refused nothing, unless it interfered with the experiment. What the questioners didn't realise was that we were feeling our way. They could not see why the Doctors didn't set up cultural and religious sections, and could not visualise that these things could come in time naturally. We had had frustrating war years, a good many of us in the prime of life, the Centre was a joyous release, so it was natural for the emphasis to be on the physical. We needed five years or more for rehabilitation, and then if we could have functioned on, we would have found out how to live, and with the richness of our talents who knows what would have happened?

The Cafeteria was already a 'bush telephone' – if help or advice was needed, it was to be found by talking to someone who would pass one on to someone else if necessary. For example, a mother entering hospital need not fear, someone would volunteer to have the children.

People came together through mutual interests – and from that came close friendships. And the young people, what a wide selection they had.

This brings me on to the Sunday afternoon or evening meetings. On the reopening of the Centre, there were no urgent requests for Sunday opening, so the Doctors found it very convenient for meetings. These arose because it was apparent that the members wanted to know what was going on. There were no long prearranged dates, but when the Doctors felt they had something to say we gathered together. I cannot remember what was said, but the idea was to keep the members informed of what was happening, and to answer members' questions. To describe these meetings is practically impossible. I am afraid of being accused of over emotionalism or sentimentality, but I will try. Firstly the attendance was almost incredible. Mum, Dad, Grandparents and teenagers, sitting around the Doctors, all completely at ease. The long room would be full – and that no small area. I can remember I would look around, and say to myself, 'I love these people.' Here was what our visitors wanted: our first spiritual manifestation.

Of course it was very apparent that the Doctors loved their families, and the families responded. There was a warm glow, nothing that one could lay ones hand upon, something indescribable, that I have never felt again.

It has been said to me by many visitors, that the Doctors were the Centre, and that without them it would not survive. I would agree that they were the loving centre of the Centre, but others could be trained. The Doctors were – to put it in my simple language 'good' people, and others can be found. I would watch for a while a new member of the staff, and say to myself quite confidently, 'He will do,' or, 'She will do.' Since the Centre closed I have always assessed life and people by Centre standards, and occasionally I have come across someone who could have functioned with the Centre.

I think I should here pay tribute to the Doctors and try to convey the love and admiration the members had for them. I never encountered a member who did not look forward to the family consultation, and who did not benefit in some way. Dr Williamson was called by most of the men 'Doc'; the women were more formal and called both Dr Williamson and Dr Pearse 'Doctor'. Doctor as spoken by a member was the sound of someone saying 'Mother' or 'Father'.

Even those members who were always wanting to turn the Centre into a paying club with an elected Committee, admitted their admiration and affection for the Doctors.

I have maintained in this writing that not many members understood the experiment – but again just a few short years (and in my summary of the work we did to try and keep the Centre open, I shall contradict this statement, with the story I have to tell).

I had helped the Doctors with visitors in the early weeks of the reopening, then with typing notes etc. Quite suddenly as the word got round throughout the UK and the world, everyone wanted to visit the Centre.

A 'Visits' Secretary was appointed, and I became her assistant, and a part-time member of staff. When not working, I reverted to being a member, and joined in a number of activities.

The Secretary or I took visitors round the Centre, and answered such questions as we were able, then, if they were lucky, they had tea with the Doctors. I say lucky, because it was impossible for the Doctors to meet everyone. Visitors came from everywhere, in ones and twos – some very VIP – or in groups from most of the women's organisations, student groups, British Council, nursing and health visitors, universities, and medical students. I must say I tried to 'duck out' from the last year medical students, I found them overbearing, sarcastic and indoctrinated. Although I would always explain that I could not answer any questions. If the work going on in the Centre penetrated through to the odd one or two, he or she would ask to come again on their own, and a number did. The Doctors were patient in the extreme with these boorish young people, and gave of their knowledge and experience without stint. I enjoyed taking round and talking to the various women's organisations they identified their families with our member families, and their most urgent question was, 'How can we get a Centre of our own?'

Before long, appointments for visits became booked for a year ahead.

Miss Moor and other members of the staff were out speaking at various organisations, and with the demand for speakers, my turn came. As far as I can recall, Miss Moor was becoming submerged, and Dr Williamson said, 'Thats all right; Elsie can do some.' I suppose I visited one or two meetings a week, either in the afternoon or evening, mostly in the Home Counties. Other members of the staff went further afield, and of course the Doctors were in constant demand.

This was a very enjoyable period for me. I revelled in the opportunity to 'spread the news' as it were. But in the end, it was too much for all of us, we became tired and harassed, and Doctor Williamson said there must be an end.

So I was allowed to circulate as one of the children's wardens (I use the word warden, but have no doubt that in time, we would have coined our own name for the person working on the social floor.) I gave 'tickets' out to the children, and kept an eye on things in general throughout the building. The children from the Centre school could be anywhere in the Centre during the afternoon and would occupy quite a bit of my time, and then after school would come the older children.

At two o'clock I would then don my swimsuit and go down to the learners' pool. A lovely little bath. Each afternoon the water started at a few inches, and rose gradually, so mothers were able to bring their babies and let them feel the water. I usually got into the pool because the children loved to splash me. They taught themselves to swim, the pattern was practically identical with all the children, first a dog paddle with one foot on the bottom, then a push from the side and a dog paddle under the water, and it could be sometimes quite a while before they found out how to surface, when they did that they were swimming and ready for the big bath. By experimenting with the water and taking their own time, they became very good swimmers and quite unafraid of the water.

How right this was – so many times I have seen youngsters struggling to learn, being bullied and coaxed by parents, and worst of all, being made to do a breast stroke, which isn't a natural stroke, all in a bath where the water is too deep. In fact it has happened in our family – Tony at ten swam like a fish, my grandson Mike is ten, and still has one foot on the bottom!

After the session in the small pool, I would circulate and quite often found myself at the piano, continuing the games etc, which we had been doing in the morning at the school. The favourite I can remember very well – the children loved to be flowers growing in a garden – loud lively music made them grow, soft music sent them to sleep.

Then as toddlers tired and mothers collected, I was available for the children coming in from school. I did an awful lot of reading, it was obvious that a number of children did not get enough stories read to them, and I would be handed a book – and a group would collect round me and sit down on the floor wherever I happened to be.

If I wasn't caught up with other things, I would join Tony and his gang in the swimming pool. Good job I was a reasonable swimmer; I had a very rough time!

I watched the Centre school being born. Just as we had insisted that the Centre must reopen. So now the parents told the Doctors they wanted a Centre school. I attended meetings as an observer – from the beginning the parents were part of the school. Administration was by the parents, and a parent with a particular skill or ability might come to the school to help.

The closing of the Centre

From the moment it was announced the Centre must close, members clamoured for action, and after the closing we were allowed the use of an old house attached to the Centre grounds. It was a couple of minutes from my home, and for some weeks I spent most of my time there. The members had decided they would continue their subscriptions as a fighting fund, and for running expenses. We had a room where members could come for a chat and cup of tea, and another where we set up an office. Hundreds of letters were written to subscribers and friends of the Centre, Members of Parliament and local councillors etc. We had hoped to enlist sympathy and help from our local MPs but none was forthcoming. We had written to all local MPs but only one responded, the late Major Vernon, from one of the Dulwich constituencies. As far as I know he had never visited the Centre, but he became our firm friend, and I shall always remember him and his kindness to us.

There were many letters of support and some money, but the support the Doctors had needed, and which we tried to get, was not forthcoming.

I am sure the answer is in my previous notes about visitors. Women's organisations, when visiting the Centre, wanted to know *how they could get a Centre of their own*. The Establishment were afraid. The Peckham Experiment could and would turn everything topsy-turvy: politicians and civil servants like comfort and would not appreciate being diverted from their accustomed courses. And then of course, there were the new 'Health' centres just being opened, although one didn't enter a health centre unless one was sick! This opinion was arrived at after meetings we had with a group of women MPs and then the Labour MPs of the London Boroughs. Of course I can't remember what was said, but I do know I was very angry, I could get no response from the women, and the London MPs were in the main very rude and abrupt. All with shut minds (deliberately?). They certainly had no intention of helping us in any way.

We had various meetings with members and staff of the London County Council, who were, I think, a little afraid of us. We should of course have been in some awe of the Council. They were a very impressive bunch. Even their Legal Department was represented, and I remember how very proud I was to be among the members representing the Centre. We stood up to a battery of questions very easily; we knew our subject!

Finally after more than one meeting, a proposition was made to us. It was this: the Centre would reopen under the auspices of the LCC but without the Doctors and the Medical Department. We questioned further and found there was no understanding of family membership. There would undoubtedly be a session for grown-ups, and others for teenagers and children. Everything would be well organised!

They could not envisage the family doing things together or apart, without the utmost chaos. So – no more table tennis with my son, Tony. Tony and his friends would never in a world of Sundays throw me into the deep end of the swimming pool. The girls and occasionally the odd boys would no longer watch their mothers machining and sewing. Our teenage girl billiards champion would no longer play with adults of similar skill, etc etc. For the children to be allowed access to all parts of the building up to six o'clock couldn't even be thought about. Their minds boggled. Or did they? That is a question that has never been answered. I had more than a feeling that, like the MPs, they didn't want the upheaval that the new concept in living would bring.

So without family membership and the Doctors, the answer from the Centre members was, 'No, – nothing doing!' (We were indeed pressed, and I had the feeling that the LCC would have been delighted if we had accepted, the Centre would have been highly publicised as another achievement by the great LCC.)

The members had further gatherings together, and we were loaned a school hall and ran for a little time a Youth Club, but it wasn't successful. Youth needs the stimulus of different age groups, and that we couldn't give them, so we shut down.

Of course we were all shattered. For most members the backbone of their lives had been taken away. I was going to say, especially those with babies and young children. That isn't right; each and every individual was affected. All of us had relied very much on the yearly overhaul and family consultation, to set our course for the coming year – to help us decide, for example, on an addition to the family, a change of job, a change of school, a school leaver's career etc, or perhaps a hidden medical fear brought into the open and dealt with. I could go on at some length with examples. All problems could be discussed so easily with the Doctors.

I have forgotten during the passing years many things, and some precious memories were put deliberately behind me, in order to go on living. But I can recall with great pleasure, and as if it were yesterday, families coming from the Medical Department, after their family consultation, into the Cafeteria for a cup of tea. They had, after perhaps their second year's overhaul, delight and happiness in their eyes and a glow around them. (This last sentence is extreme, I know, and is one of the reasons why, after many attempts, I have given up trying to write about the Centre; it is extremely difficult, impossible almost, to describe these experiences without being accused of over indulgence and sentimentality, *but* – glow they did!) How can I explain that we knew what was going on around us – I suppose it really was very simple – a cup of tea here, a word there, we all knew and liked each other, so it was no hardship to say, 'I'm having my overhaul this afternoon,' or, 'We have our family consultation this evening, when are you having yours?' Our lives were very much interlinked.

From a practical point of view some of us were in trouble. We had been used to quite a deal of physical exercise, and needed to go on with this. So a friend and I decided we would have to go to evening classes.

We returned to the Centre building, which had been taken over by the LCC.

We needed courage to do this, and it wasn't very nice; the interior of the building had been altered, the cafeteria closed right in, everything and everywhere was quiet, no fun or laughter or chatter. I felt as if I should walk on tip toe. And, I had to face the formidable Area Principal, whom we had met on her visits to the Centre when it was functioning; she could not or would not understand and was continually 'tut-tutting'. We had suffered her sarcastic remarks on many occasions, and here she was triumphant; she had the Centre building for her own. How she would have liked to have had the Centre members as well!

We joined the Old Tyme dancing class, which wasn't too bad, if we kept our minds on the dancing. One little incident sticks in my mind. A teenager came and stood behind one of the pillars watching the class. He was doing no harm at all, but the Area Principal came along, and the teenager was told off and made to look small. Had it been Centre days, he would have been nicely ignored, or smiled at, and he could have watched at any time he liked. We know of course that it was one of the ways in which so many members first interested themselves in the various activities.

We had to join a swimming class, otherwise we couldn't use the pool; so we did. I think that lasted about three evenings, we were so bored. We didn't want at our age to compete in the Olympics – just to swim – but, as soon as we fell out of line, we were told to get into place.

I didn't stay very long at the evening classes; the atmosphere was depressing, and there were too many ghosts.

In conclusion, two four-year periods was all we had; we had only just begun to grow in health.

For me personally, the closing of the Centre was real heartbreak – for I wanted passionately to see the children grow and flower, and perhaps their children, which of course I could have done had things not gone wrong.

Not only were the two Doctors growing health with wholeness, but love in the true sense of the word.

Elsie Purser

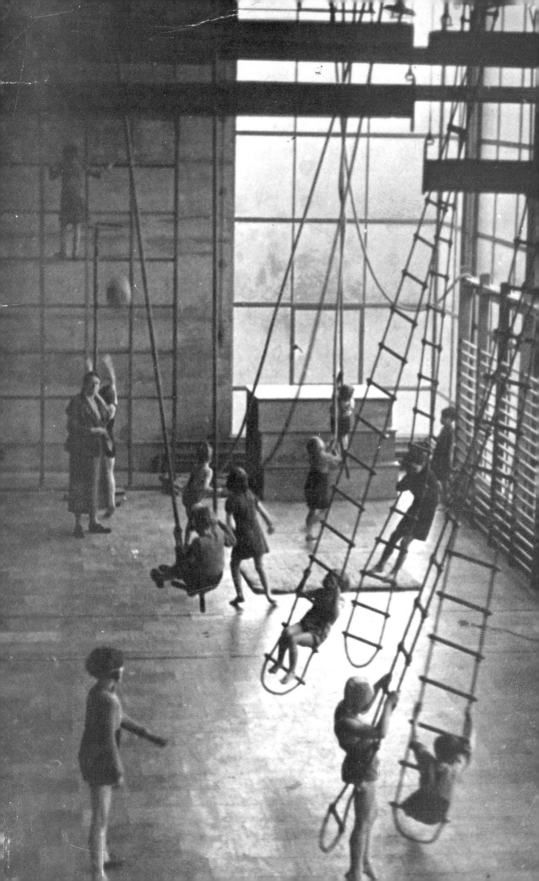

Part Three

The Growth of Freedom and Responsibility

Chapter 9

The Biological Laws Governing Child Development

The contribution of Jean Piaget

Jean Piaget has been called the giant of developmental psychology; yet I fear it may not be long before people begin to wonder why. This is because his greatest gift to posterity, his theory of how a baby's mental faculties grow, how he learns the nature of his surroundings and how to be effective in them is almost entirely ignored.

By great good fortune, the first of his books that I came across was *The Origin of Intelligence in the Child* which contains the essence of this theory. I realised with excitement that his thought ran on similar lines to that of Scott Williamson, and, eventually, that their two theories of how a child's faculties develop were basically the same. Probably my experience of the Centre had made me capable of appreciating Piaget's theory, but, having studied it thoroughly, I was able to understand better what Scott Williamson meant by 'the faculty for choice' and the 'subjective synthesis of experience.'

Piaget was fascinated with natural history from childhood. As a schoolboy, he spent his Saturdays helping a zoologist with his research into the effect of different habitats on the body shape of a certain fresh water mollusc. He remained a biologist in outlook throughout his long career as a philosopher and psychologist.

The Origin of Intelligence in the Child was first published in French in 1936. Therefore Piaget was working on his theory of how a baby comes to know and think and develop mentally and functionally at about the same time as Scott Williamson was developing his awareness of the biological facts of mental and functional growth.

Considerable application is required to follow Piaget's argument partly because he compares it, at every stage, with theories already propounded on the subject. But throughout he illustrates it with hundreds of 'observations' selected from the voluminous diaries in which he had recorded on the spot the behaviour of his own three children from birth until the age of two or three. The observations are written in simple and vivid language and, from them and his comments on them, it is easy to obtain a clear understanding of his thought. This lengthy and intensive piece of observational research together with the little experiments he did with the children constitute by far the most important piece of ethological research on human infants in their familiar home environment that has ever been carried out. In fact there has been little competition. The only writer who has devoted any considerable length of time to the observation of the entirely spontaneous behaviour of a baby is the American biologist, Milicent Washburn Shinn.* She studied the spontaneous behaviour of her niece during the first year of life with a truly open and enquiring mind, and, like Piaget, with a respect for the subject of her study that is characteristic of present-day students of animal behaviour. Her findings corroborate those of Piaget. I have quoted her at length in *The Self-Respecting Child*.†

Piaget's theory of how intelligence develops

Piaget looked at human beings with the same respect and wonder that he had felt for water snails. He did not split them, either the snails or the children, into bodies on the one hand and minds on the other. So it did not surprise him to find that babies spontaneously grow intellectually, as well as physically. The problem was *how*. How, he wondered, does the almost completely helpless new-born infant become a capable two year old?

He asked himself such questions as, 'Why did Lucienne suck her fingers, a quarter of an hour after birth, for ten minutes in succession?' And comments. 'It could not be because of hunger because the umbilical cord had only just been cut.' It could not have been comforting to her, as sucking a finger or thumb might later become, because her efforts were so clumsy and unskilled. That she should begin to suck at her hand was to be expected for it was held closely against her mouth owing to the manner in which she had been wrapped up, and the 'sucking reflex' (or tendency to make sucking movements at a touch on the open mouth) would have come into play automatically. But, Piaget asks, 'Why did she continue to suck for so long when sucking led to no apparent result?' His answer is that Lucienne was practising sucking. Her faculty to suck was beginning to develop through being exercised on something. Sneezing and blinking are – and remain – automatic 'reflex' reactions to stimuli but sucking begins as a reflex action which, as soon as it is used on an object, changes to become an organised whole capable of growth and differentiation. What happens is that the presence of a thumb in a baby's mouth triggers off mechanical sucking movements. These are energetic but inept. However, after a few moments, if the thumb remains in his mouth, the baby's lips and tongue begin to shape themselves to the thumb, and his sucking movements begin to accommodate themselves to its form and consistency. Little by little the inborn ability to make sucking movements develops into a faculty-to-suck-a-thumb. The baby continues automatically to suck at anything that falls into his mouth, but, if it happens to be a thumb, his faculty-to-suck-a-thumb operates

* 1900, republished 1988
† 1974

immediately at its existing stage of efficiency. The baby does not have to learn from scratch on each occasion; he begins almost exactly where he left off, and soon the specific movements of his cheeks, jaws and tongue that are necessary for the effective sucking of a thumb will have become co-ordinated in space and time and organised to form a whole that is called into play in its entirety whenever his thumb finds its way into his mouth. If the circumstances are different – if, for instance, a baby finds a different object such as a nipple or a dummy or a piece of his clothing in his mouth – he may, in the first moment, make use of his faculty-to-suck-a-thumb upon the new object, and then adapt it to the new circumstances. This happens without causing the knowledge of how to suck a thumb to be erased from his memory. Henceforth the baby's faculty to suck or, as Piaget calls it, the baby's 'sucking schema' now consists of several distinct skills, one of which is called into play by the sensation of a thumb in his mouth, another by a nipple, a third by a dummy and a fourth by a fold of material. His sucking schema requires to be exercised on a variety of objects if it is to differentiate in this manner; it needs what Piaget calls 'aliment':

> The object sucked is to be conceived, not as nourishment for the organism in general, but, so to speak, as aliment for the very activity of sucking.*

In other words, the schema needs to nourish itself on the environment. And, given the chance, it does. Although Lucienne had taken her first breath only fifteen minutes earlier and so did not feel hungry for milk, she already had an appetite for the kind of experience that would nourish her faculty to suck.

Then the sucking schema branches out; it differentiates still further; new shoots grow from the main stem. At 30 days old, Piaget's son Laurent lies making rhythmical sucking movements. 'At certain moments, his tongue, instead of remaining inside his lips, licks the lower lip.' Then:

> Observation 12. At 0:1(3) [One month and three days], Laurent puts out his tongue several times in succession. He is wide awake, motionless, hardly moves his arms and makes no sucking-like movements; his mouth is partly open and he keeps passing his tongue over his lower lip. At 0:1(5) Laurent begins sucking-like movements and then the sucking is gradually replaced by the preceding behaviour. At 1:1(6) he plays with his tongue, sometimes licking his lower lip, sometimes sliding his tongue between his lips and gums. The following days this behaviour is frequently repeated and always with the same expression of satisfaction.†

The sucking schema is adapting itself to new situations and thus extends itself; and at the same time, it is assimilating new items of knowledge and knowhow into itself. The result is a new schema, 'the exploring-with-the-tongue-schema'.

---

* 1936
† *ibid.*

At this time, the baby's seeing schema (or faculty to see) is also beginning to grow through exercising itself on the environment.

At 30 days old, Laurent:

> ... stares at a piece of fringe on his cradle with continuous little re-adaptive movements as though his head had difficulty in not changing position, and his gaze brought it to the right place again. So long as he gazes thus, his arms are still; at other times when he is awake, they tend to wave to and fro.

Piaget says that the activity of looking at something nourishes the child's faculty to see.

In this, (as in the previous 'observation') there is evidence that the baby is attending to what is happening. At that moment, the baby's whole being is affected by the fact that he is engaged in developing the physical and mental processes that are involved in seeing, and this causes the temporary inhibition of the almost continuous involuntary movements of the arms that a baby of this age makes when awake. At this age, the infant's ability to keep objects in focus, to use both eyes together and to direct and control the movements of his eyeballs is ready to develop rapidly if exercised. 'Almost from birth,' Piaget says, 'there is 'behaviour' in the sense of the individual's total reaction, and not only a setting in motion of particular or local automatizations.'

In the large section on grasping, Piaget noted of Laurent that:

> At 0:2(7) [two months and seven days] he scratches the sheet which is folded over the blankets, then grasps it and holds it a moment, lets it go, then scratches it again and grasps it, and so on without interruption. At 0:2(11) this play lasts a quarter of an hour at a time, several times during the day.

As Piaget explains, if a baby of this age is free to do so, he spends much of his time, when awake, waving his arms jerkily and at random and stretching and bending his fingers. He also automatically closes his fingers over an object that touches the palm of his hand or the inside of his fingers; (as most people know, he has a surprisingly strong grip at this early age). Because of these two tendencies, a baby will frequently close his fingers on his clothes or his blanket. But, under the age of two months or so, the natural tendency of the baby's hand is to jerk away again and move in some other direction. Therefore when, on the occasion described, Laurent's hand remains more or less on one spot, scratching at and momentarily holding the sheet over and over again, it seems to Piaget that Laurent is beginning to pay attention to the sensory impressions that the activity of touching the sheet gives him. He is giving evidence of the beginning of a 'tactile interest' in his environment.

During the following weeks, Piaget noticed that Laurent spent less and less time scratching, and often grasped the sheet almost on first touching it, and that he held on for longer. At this stage, Laurent's faculty to grasp is exercising itself, but only in a primitive and inept manner: he uses his fingers together as a unit and his thumb with them instead of opposite to them. Therefore it is only if he encounters something which fits easily into the palm of his hand or which, like a sheet, moulds itself to his hand, that he can hold it.

At $2^1/_2$ months, Laurent is grasping at all sorts of things, still in a hit and miss manner because his actions tend to be undiscriminating: he is using a similar movement of his fingers on every occasion, whatever the shape and consistency of the object. But then it sometimes happens that, before he relaxes his grip or stretches his fingers again after having closed them upon an object, he has received something from the object. This something is a bit of knowledge of how to grasp that particular object. It is evident that the baby retains and absorbs this bit of sensory-motor knowledge, because, as he grasps at his sheet, or his own hand or his nose again and again, he begins to adapt the manner in which he holds and moves his fingers and thumb according to which of the objects it is that he is grasping. He begins to shape his hand to the shape of the object and to move his fingers and thumb in a manner that suits its consistency and weight.

These are instances of the interaction between the baby and his environment which, Piaget says, is the essence of mental life. It consists – in his terms – of the simultaneous assimilation of the environment by the schema and the accommodation of the schema to the environment and results in the adaptation (or reorganisation and development) of the schema. One could put it that the child's body of knowhow grows by digesting selected experiences of the environment while at the same time adapting itself to the reality of the environment or, more vividly, as Drusilla Scott has done:

> A schema absorbs the new into what is already there, modifies what is already there to accommodate the new and so keeps the baby's knowledge growing.*

If one thinks of what is happening when one is acquiring a practical skill, it is evident that the skill grows by being exercised in a manner that is more and more finely atuned to the needs of the situation in which it is being used: it is accommodating itself to reality. It also grows by being used in an increasing variety of situations: the skill is assimilating the new environmental circumstances to itself and thus is extending itself. Piaget's observational research has shown that a baby's essential human abilities begin very early to grow in this manner, and that the baby instinctively acts on his environment in a way that enables them to do so. For instance, he exercises his grasping and holding ability on the same objects over and over again, so that it gradually increases. An

* 1985

observer will notice that certain objects are becoming known to the baby as objects to be grasped in a particular manner. On encountering them, he more often quickly makes the appropriate movements of his fingers and hands; he fumbles and experiments less, until eventually, at the first touch of one of them, he may immediately make the precise movements that are necessary in order to take hold of it effectively. He also attempts to grasp and hold an increasing variety of objects.

D O Hebb in *A Textbook of Psychology* writes that a healthy baby is interested in things that are intriguingly new but that have a certain similarity to things with which he is already familiar, things that are different but not too different, things that have a quality of 'difference-in-sameness'. Piaget puts it that the baby pays attention to that in his environment which one of his schemata is, at the moment, capable of assimilating to itself and accommodating itself to. (Compare this with the Peckham Biologists' 'appetitive phases'.)

In all of this activity, the baby's discriminating and directing intelligence is at work; his body and mind are working together as a whole, and he himself is directing the work of the whole; he is building up a body of knowledge and knowhow.

Piaget's discussion on the difference in value between learning through imitation that is undertaken spontaneously by the child and being trained to imitate is very interesting in view of the Peckham Biologists' experience and opinions regarding training.* Imitation secured by the repeated reinforcement of a conditioned association he calls 'pseudo-imitation'; real imitation is the result of 'assimilation'. He says that the most obvious difference between the two is that pseudo-imitation does not last: the power to imitate a certain movement is soon lost if the training is interrupted. This is because the baby does not at this stage possess a body-of-knowledge and knowhow into which this particular bit of knowhow can be incorporated. Another difference between skills acquired by training and those acquired by digestion because the baby is ready and eager to learn them is that the latter are adaptable to new circumstances; they are living and capable of growth.

The argument for 'training' as an aid to performance in small children is usually ranged against the theory that anatomical maturation is all-important, at least for the acquisition of motor skills involving the whole body. In these discussions, no distinction is made between training and spontaneous practice as, for example, in Gessell's often-quoted experiment with identical twins and stair-climbing.†

In *The Self-Respecting Child*, I have given an account of Piaget's observations of how the babies continued to create their intellectual and sensory-motor powers, of how one faculty developed from another or from the 'mutual assimilation' of two 'schemas', of how babies, as he says, 'tend to behave like scientists – to experiment in order to see', and

* See Chapter 10, p. 264
† See *The Self-Respecting Child*, Chapter 7

of how they begin to solve practical problems intellectually (in their heads) instead of using a slow trial and error method. He shows how they do this by bringing to bear on the problem a combination of bits of previously digested knowledge or knowhow. He says that the 'invention of new means through mental combinations' is not different in essence from the activity of a baby when he combines his grasping schema and his reaching-for schema and his judging-the-distance-in-space-of-an-object schema in order to retrieve a toy from the foot of his pram. He records many instances of both the slow trial and error method and the quicker, entirely mental method of solving the problems that his children came upon in their play or were set up by himself. After the age of about fifteen months, they sometimes used the slow method of practical experiment and sometimes solved them 'in their heads'.

Piaget's descriptions contain evidence of the joy that their spontaneous learning-activities gave the children, even as young as four months, e.g. 'laughs uproariously at the results obtained'; 'repeats the action several times with much laughter'; or 'smiles broadly while wriggling and kicking with pleasure'.

I remember an instance of a baby enjoying being effective. We were in a restaurant in Brittany. A family at the next table were enjoying a lengthy Sunday dinner. A baby of about a year was perched in a high chair next to her father. He was indefatigably keeping her from getting bored. I noticed that the behaviour on his part that made her happiest was when he responded to some action on her part with some exaggerated grimace or gesture and repeated the response every time she repeated the action.

The implications of Piaget's theory

On reading *The Origin of Intelligence in the Child*, two questions spring to mind: (1) If a child's intellectual and sensory-motor knowledge and effectiveness grow in this way during his first year, will they not continue to grow in the same way – his material and human environment permitting – throughout his childhood and his whole life, and, in growing, continue to give him joy? (2) If early intellectual ability and sensory-motor judgment grow in this way, why not also other human faculties such as the form of judgment that is called wisdom, or responsibility for oneself and one's surroundings, or the ability to form and maintain mutually enjoyable relationships with others.

Robert Winthrop White, Professor Emeritus of Clinical Psychology at Harvard University, throws light on these questions in his *Motivation Reconsidered: the concept of competence.** This paper is written in lucid and jargon-free English and is a joy to read. He is one of the few psychologists who have fully understood the vitally important implications of Piaget's work on how children develop mentally.

* 1959

Piaget asked how babies learn; Robert White asked why. His theory of motivation is well documented; he himself describes it as a 'gathering together' of ideas that have been stated in one way or another by workers in many different branches of psychology and biology and belonging to differing schools of thought. These people have stated their dissatisfaction with the hitherto generally accepted theories of motivation, such as the one that attributes activity to the need to reduce the tension caused by somatic 'drives', or to habits formed through tension having been reduced in the past. They have postulated an 'instinct to master', an 'exploratory instinct', a 'Functionslust', 'autonomous ego development', or observed a tendency 'to act so as to produce an optimum level of stimulation in the environment'.*

White describes how students of animal behaviour have, time and again, observed that animals do not need the prospect of a reward to push them into investigating new objects, exploring new territory and learning new skills; monkeys will work for weeks at solving simple mechanical puzzles with no reward other than finding a solution; and 'even rats enjoy solving problems when all their sensual needs have been purposely sated.' One researcher reported that rats would cross an electrified grill simply for the privilege of exploring further afield; and, in fact, it was found that hungry rats do not solve difficult problems, the solution of which is rewarded by food, as effectively as rats that are not particularly hungry; the reason being that the former are in so much of a hurry to reach the food that they do not take into account all the factors necessary to the solution of the problem.

Robert White holds that it is important to 'conceptualize the principle behind these independently stated results of research and thought because their very vital common properties have been lost to view amidst the strongly analytical tendencies that go with detailed research,' for together they amount to 'a significant evolution of ideas concerning what it is that motivates animals and human beings to act.'†

He says that the child's need for food, sleep and cuddling demands immediate satisfaction when it occurs, but it occurs only intermittently; the very strong desires the child feels for these things interrupt from time to time the more gentle but steady and persistent urge he feels to develop his powers and to make himself familiar with his environment.

He observes that the play of babies is not 'random behaviour produced by a general overflow of energy' nor are they at the mercy of any and every stimulus; on the contrary, 'their behaviour is directed, selective and persistent.'¶

He puts it that the purposeful efforts of children to learn to see, grasp, walk, think and speak – and of all young mammals to make themselves

---

* 1959
† *ibid.*
¶ *ibid.*

familiar with their environment and to exercise their faculties – have a common biological significance: they are the result of the need to become 'competent', that is to say, to become 'capable of interacting effectively with the environment'. The playing child does not know that he must exercise his faculties in order to become a competent human being; he does so because he enjoys it, and he enjoys it because it gives him a sense of power over himself and circumstances. It reinforces his feeling of possessing the ability to respond to his surroundings as he would like to respond to them. White puts it that behaviour which promotes the development of latent ability in any field of activity gives an animal or a human being a satisfying 'feeling of efficacy'. He main-tains that Piaget's research and that of animal ethologists points to the conclusion that young creatures are motivated by an urge to do that which leads, eventually, to their becoming competent people, tigers, badgers, otters or whatever. (This is not the same thing as saying that they practise the skills they will need as adults. In the case of infants-in-arms, this would be nonsense.)

White points out that this view of motivation makes evolutionary sense: individuals possessing an especially strong urge to develop their potential powers and to relate effectively with their environment would have been the most likely to survive and reproduce.

In another book, he writes:

A person's conception of himself is nourished partly by the way others treat him and the things they say about him but the heart of his self-feeling is in what he feels able to do.*

Children need to feel that they are lovable, but also to feel confident of being able to act in a manner that they consider competent.

Robert White's theory of motivation is little known in Britain; and, in the country in which he has lived and worked, although he is respected as a teacher and a writer of general textbooks on psychology, attempts have been made to hide his theory of motivation with a smoke-screen of obscure verbiage or to damn it with faint praise whenever it has been impossible to ignore it.

White's theory complements Piaget's and, together with the findings of the Peckham Biologists, gives us confidence that children will continue to take the available opportunities to exercise their faculties, to acquire the knowledge and knowhow that increases their human competence, to experience what they need to experience in order to become rounded, whole, mature people, as long as the opportunities are continuously available to them. They give us confidence that the two questions posed above may be answered in the affirmative. The questions were: (1) If a child's intellectual and sensory-motor knowledge and effectiveness grow in this way during his first year, will they not continue

* 1972

to grow in the same way – his material and human environment permitting – throughout his childhood and his whole life, and, in growing, continue to give him joy? (2) If early intellectual ability and sensory-motor judgment grow in this way, why not also other human faculties such as the form of judgment that is called wisdom, or responsibility for oneself and one's surroundings, or the ability to form and maintain mutually enjoyable relationships with others?

It is necessary however, that the child's faith in his ability to grow in competence and effectiveness remains strong. Therefore, the opportunities for experience and activity available to him must be of a kind that will increase his competence *as he sees competence*. They should be of a kind that are attractive to him at the stage he has reached and they must be continuously available, not merely once a week, or at weekends or on holidays. Reading and writing and the other skills and knowledge that are a necessary part of our twentieth century culture may be attractive to him only if the people he loves and admires practise them with enjoyment, or if and when he understands that they are necessary to adult competence. But it stands to reason that confidence in his power to learn what he wants to learn (which can only come through experience) will stand him in good stead when he is subjected to formal education or begins to undergo instruction of any kind.

Piaget has said that a person's intelligence has a pre-determined limit but that this limit is very rarely ever reached. It is safe to guess that a person's potential capability as a whole, including his ability to relate effectively and wisely with his material and human environment, is rarely fully realised. If, from birth onwards, a child's environment were to be of a kind that enabled him to develop a satisfyingly effective relationship with it, would the situation be improved? If so, one must find out what sort of skills and powers children in general want to develop and make it possible for them to do so.

Perhaps the first power a child enjoys, if he is allowed to do so, is the power to find his mother's body close at hand when he wants it, to touch and cling to it, nestle against it, and to find the nipple and make the milk come by sucking. Later he enjoys finding that he can obtain a response from his mother, and then the particular response he intends at that moment to obtain. He goes on to take advantage of opportunities for obtaining sensory-motor, mental and social skills and powers, one after the other – or simultaneously.

Now that 'doorstep play' with the neighbouring toddlers is no longer possible, and impromptu games on the common or by the roadside on the way home from school rarely fall to the lot of the older child, it is absolutely essential that all the adults who are in charge of children during the day, both in school and out of it, and everyone that has any responsibility for the environment of children should understand the laws that govern healthy growth and should knowhow to provide an environment in which these laws can operate.

It is a pity that Piaget did not announce loudly and emphatically and at frequent intervals during the last forty years of his life what his findings concerning the manner in which ability grows imply, namely that the child must have the opportunity to select for himself the mental, emotional and functional nourishment he needs, to digest it in his own time, and to find, for himself, problems to solve, games to invent, challenges to meet, dreams to dream, hazards to circumvent, difficulties to overcome and friends to make and keep. If he had done so and if Robert White's theory had been enthusiastically welcomed by psychologists and educationalists and given all possible publicity, then people might have become aware of the heaven-sent opportunity that parents, nursery nurses, teachers, architects and planners have to further the happiness and mental, physical and emotional health of children.

It is also a sad thing for mankind that Jan Christian Smuts' insight into the essential characteristics of living organisms in contrast to those of inorganic matter (or aggregates of purely physical and chemical matter) has failed to influence the course of developmental psychology.

> External environmental influences are merely the rough material with which an organism works and builds up its own system. And in the act of building, the material itself is more or less completely changed into the character of the structure built.*

And that it is not in the nature of a living being to be passive in its relations with its environment. When an external cause acts on an organism, the resultant response is not the passive effect of the stimulus or cause as would be the case with a piece of inorganic material.

> The cause or stimulus applied does not issue in its own passive effect, but in an active response which seems more clearly traceable to the organism itself. In fact the physical character or 'cause' undergoes a far-reaching change in its application to organisms or wholes generally. The whole (organism) appears as the real cause of the response, and not the external stimulus, which seems to play the quite minor role of a mere excitant or condition.

The external cause or stimulus is internalised and transformed by the organism. The latter's response is to this transformed stimulus. Apart from this, if everybody perceives and experiences the environment differently, as recent investigators avow, each person's response to a particular cause is likely to be different and possibly unique. Smuts says:

> If the concept of causation is to be retained in connection with organic or psychical activities, it will have to be substantially recast. The resultant activity of an organism under a stimulus is never merely the effect of that

* Smuts, 1926. Smuts was a botanist as well as a soldier and statesman.

stimulus, as it would be in the case of mechanical action, but always of the stimulus as transformed by the organism.

This, it seems to me, is common sense. And, whatever may be true of other sciences, the propositions of biologists (and psychologists) must surely make sense to people. To be judged valid, they must conform to experience, to people's experience of life and of others' lives.

It seems to me that if biologists and psychologists had paid attention to Piaget and Robert White and to the discoveries of animal ethologists, whole university departments would have been saved a great deal of time and money, and many students might have avoided the enforced suspension of their critical faculties and the smothering of their common sense. Moreover, the sterile 'mechanism versus vitalism' and 'nature versus nurture' arguments could have been well and truly buried, instead of being resurrected at intervals and hammered away at to the waste of everybody's time.

If Piaget and White are right, a child is not something that must be manipulated, moulded and prodded into action, if he is to become a mature adult, or, indeed, that can be formed into what one would like – unless this be a robot or a slave, but is a living being which grows because it is its raison d'être to grow, and which, like a flower or a tree, knows how to grow.

The course of history

There was a time, about 20 years ago, when the English state Infant and Junior schools (ages five to eleven) acquired a world-wide reputation for being places where all children – not only the cleverest – enjoyed the school day from beginning to end, where their curiosity and appetite for knowledge were sharpened and where they were able to develop their talent for creativity, initiative, judgment and spontaneous co-operation. When this reputation was at its height, a sudden panic arose and spread as a result of the publication of figures showing a high number of illiterate school leavers. Parents became worried and some of the teachers' employers, the Local Education Authorities, began to deprive head teachers of their responsibility for the curriculum and the organisation of the children's day and to institute frequent testing on the American model. Head teachers who had fought a long and hard battle to give the children greater initiative and responsibility in the learning process and the opportunity to assimilate new knowledge and skill into their existing bodies of knowledge and knowhow and thus digest it thoroughly have been forced to toe the line – or to retire.

At the same period it became known that many children were entering school at five years old barely able to speak their mother tongue and with such small vocabularies that it was impossible to teach them to read without first teaching them to talk. It was felt that preventative measures must be taken. In nursery schools and playgroups the slogan 'Talk to the Children' was pasted up. This and the desire to prepare children for school had the effect of producing behaviour on the part of nursery supervisors such as I observed on one occasion when visiting a playgroup. A small child had made a winding, zigzag track on the floor with some long narrow pieces of plywood of different lengths laid end to end and was balancing along it, again and again, walking a little faster each time. An adult came up and said, 'Look! this piece is longer than that one. Do you think this one over here is shorter?' The child paused a moment and then resumed her game. It seems to me that a better slogan would have been 'Listen to the children'.

It has been said that Piaget formed the main opposition to the behaviourist tradition, but it is a tragic fact that, either by accident or design, his biggest guns have been spiked, and the behaviourists left in possession of the field. Evidence of this is that almost all living academic developmental psychologists appear to hold the opinion – for which they do not consider it necessary to produce any evidence – that a child will never do or learn anything of value to himself, unless he is more or less gently prodded and then rewarded with smiles and praise by attendant adults, and that his opinion of himself is entirely dependent on other people's. They are either avowed or unconscious behaviourists. An example of the former kind is, 'Attributing play to some internal intangible factor discourages a search for observable determining conditions, thereby delaying our understanding of this behaviour.'[*] The author goes on to quote someone as saying that 'a puppy chasing a rolling ball is an excellent example of generalised response to small moving objects.' I wonder if this person happened to be looking the other way when the puppy pounced on a stationary ball, thus making it into an object for chasing? In a text book for students of developmental psychology is found the following:

> The scientific study of children has appeared to have two somewhat different goals: to describe behaviour and development and to explain them... But there is no important difference between these goals... Behaviour is explained by describing it relative to other factors or environmental events.
>
> When a psychologist claims to understand behaviour, or to explain it, this means that the *determinants* (causes) of that behaviour have been identified. The two methods used to confirm the explanation are prediction and control. If the determinants of the behaviour are actually known, the scientist should be able to predict the occurrence or nonoccurrence of the behaviour by noting whether the necessary conditions exist. Likewise, the scientist should be able to control the occurrence or nonoccurrence of the behaviour by presenting or removing the necessary conditions. When these criteria are met, the scientist has explained the behaviour according to the requirements of the scientific method...[†]

[*] Bijou, 1976
[†] Vasta, 1979

Researchers belonging to this school of thought can learn only very superficial (and often dangerously misleading) things about human nature.

Some developmental psychologists have been particularly concerned to find ways of helping 'culturally disadvantaged children'. Perhaps this predisposed them to adhere to behaviourism with its emphasis on teaching rather than learning and its concentration on looking for more effective methods of controlling the children's mental behaviour. Professor Jerome Bruner wrote, with his fellow editor in the concluding chapter of *The Growth of Competence**:

> The question arose of how one may best 'manage' the period of immaturity, how shall it be used to equip the growing child with the wherewithal in skills to get on in a complex culture. One is faced immediately not only with the task of analysing how in fact the period of immaturity is used in different species of the primate order, but (in the case of man) how one *should* use it. For it is characteristic of man that he in fact must create the patterns of behaviour that suit the very environmental conditions which he has also created. Man lives in a man-made world by shaping behaviour appropriate to it, or if not shaping it, predisposing it in certain ways...
>
> We are possibly approaching then, a new period in world history where we shall have to think how to give aid and support to the family, to the child through other supportive institutions as well, and in so doing, we shall have to think afresh what kind of human beings we want. How to use the years of growth for instilling the requisite forms of competence.

A number of unacknowledged assumptions underlie these statements and the chapter in which they are found:

1. That members of the species man are psychologically – if not physically – infinitely adaptable.

2. That it is possible for mankind to come to a decision as to the kind of human beings they want.

3. That it is possible, by a process of trial and error, to discover techniques of shaping young human beings so that when adult they will be 'the kind of human beings we want'.

4. That the most important kinds of competence are those that enable a person to cope with the particular environmental conditions that obtain in our 'man-made world'.

Later Bruner and Connolly add, with regard to the young that are caught in the poverty cycle,

> Much of the problem has to do with how one instils a feeling of being in control of one's destiny, rather than feeling a victim.

* 1972

It is true that to enable a child to feel that he can be to some extent in control of his fate should be one of the aims of education; but it seems to me that the writers have no understanding of how to do this. Surely, it would not enhance a person's self-respect and sense of autonomy to feel that he is at the receiving end of a process in which people are trying to instil the requisite forms of competence or feelings into him. It seems to me that Bruner and Connolly ignore certain indisputable facts of life such as that it is impossible to teach a person wisdom or any kind of judgement – although they can be learned; impossible to instil percep- tiveness of reality into a person or creative originality or responsibility, initiative, perseverence, resilience, curiosity, strength of will and feeling, joyfulness, serenity, grace or the primitive forms of human competence dear to the hearts of children, such as sensory-motor co-ordination or the ability to balance perfectly while moving. They are unaware also that the only possible way to promote faculties and qualities such as these in a child, is to provide him with the kind of physical and social environment that allows him to exercise – and thus develop – them as far as his potentiality for them goes.

The import of what Bruner and Connolly are saying to their fellow psychologists is that it is both preferable and easier to adapt young human beings to fit the environmental conditions that man has created than to adapt these conditions to suit the needs of growing human beings, and that it is therefore quite unnecessary to try to find out what these needs are.

Although these psychologists do not admit that they adhere to the behaviourist school of thought, they must, I think, have been influenced by it. Another example is provided by the editors of *Developmental Psychology* (1975). Although in their introduction, J Sants and H J Butcher affirm the enormous debt that psychology owes to Piaget, they have included a paper by J Kagan, headed 'The Determinants of Atten- tion *in the Infant*' [my emphasis] that ends with the statement, 'The central problem in educating children is to maintain focussed attention.' This may be the central problem for teachers as lecturers but nothing could be more completely contrary to Piaget's theory of how children learn.

It is true that therapy needs to be applied to children who have suffered badly from the effects of an inadequate and sick environment. For instance, children who have not found verbal communication with other people an agreeable experience may need a great deal of skilled help and encouragement if they are to learn to speak their mother tongue and therefore to be able to learn to read. But to treat all children as if they were sick is to prevent them from being healthy.

Perhaps there should be two distinct departments of developmental psychology in universities, one working to devise therapeutic environments for disadvantaged children and the other concerned to discover the developmental needs of healthy children.

Both should, in my view, avoid concentrating on the development of intellectual skills, especially in the very young. Professor Bruner set up the Oxford Pre-School Research Group in 1975. The group's aim was 'to find out how to make knowledge about early human development of practical use to those concerned with the care of the pre-school young',* and to 'study the behaviour of children in playgroups and nursery schools'.† But judging from thier periodic newsletter, they concentrated more and more on the behaviour of the teachers and the effect of this on the children. They tried to find out

> ... how far they [the children] are being encouraged to develop concen-
> tration (an essential attribute of a competent schoolchild), how far
> language development is positively encouraged and so on.¶

Kathy Sylva, the author of one of the OPRG publications, *Child Watching in Playgroup and Nursery School*, wrote, 'As researchers... we decided to look directly at cognitive stretch.' They divided play into two categories – 'complex or high level of challenge play and ordinary play'. The first was also termed 'rich' play and was found to be either 'sequentially organised and elaborated or contained symbolic transformation' or both. The OPRG as a whole tended to value intellectual activity over any other, and to view the purpose of nursery schools and playgroups as training grounds for school. They hoped to 'identify different strategies that [nursery] teachers use in getting across skills, attitudes and values' and pass them on to others. Among these people, there appeared to be no appreciation of the value of a child's unique individuality and potential creativity, and no recognition of the universal instinct to acquire skills – both those that are specific to the human species and those that are specific to the culture which the child is born into.

A perusal of the books in the Developmental Psychology section of the library of the Institute of Education in London leads one to conclude that their authors take it for granted that a person's character and ability are entirely the result of what has been done to him by people and circumstances. (The only exceptions are the one or two who state vehemently that the genes have the major effect; but they too think of a person as being the passive victim of his fate – in this case his heredity.) From this belief it follows that the caretakers of children are in duty bound to spend every available minute stimulating children and gently steering them into activity that, it is hoped, will develop their mental ability; it follows that it is wrong merely to let them be.

In my search through the shelves at the London University Institute of Education, I came on only one refreshing breath of common sense: in *What is a Child*, N Tucker says:

---

* OPRG Newsletter No. 1, October 1975
† *ibid.*
¶ OPRG Newsletter No. 3, September 1976

Surely it is a fact that the more often children have to live in a man-made environment, the more necessary it is for parents and the planners and creators of this environment to be aware of how and in what circumstances healthy human growth occurs.

There is still room for research into the best methods of enabling children to acquire cultural skills. Piaget's work has inspired some important innovations in the field of mathematics, especially in Infant and Junior schools. Various kinds of structural apparatus have been devised, the use of which enables children to understand the basic arithmetical processes and relationships and simple algebraic equations through the use of their visual and tactile senses. The Colour Factor apparatus was used throughout one Infant School in Croydon[*], Surrey, from which, over a number of years, no child went on to a Junior School with a distaste for maths or a conviction that he was 'bad at it'.

However, what is needed above all else is knowledge of how to provide the circumstances in which children may achieve what Scott Williamson called 'facultisation'. He held that a child must be allowed to develop the basic faculties of a human being before being expected to become a cultured one. A child who has the opportunity to admire cultured, literate and numerate people will probably want to acquire similar skills himself, but he is still more likely to do so if he has the feeling of worth and the confidence that the possession of the basic human faculties has given him. A child who has developed the kind of physical, mental and social ability that has been important to human beings during the hundreds of thousands of years they have been on the earth is likely to want to go on to develop the abilities necessary for effective participation in the activities prevalent in the particular human culture to which he belongs.

One of the harmful effects of the prevailing academic view is that many parents, influenced by the consensus of opinion in the universities, feel overwhelmed by their responsibility. They feel unequal to the task of providing all the necessary input. So, they tend to decide that it is in the child's best interests, as well as to their own convenience, to hand him over to professional caretakers and teachers as early as possible. When they do keep the little one by them, they tend to be so preoccupied with worry about what they ought to be doing to him that they are unable to be responsive to the needs and desires that he is trying to communicate to them, and unable to relax in wonder and to share his joy in being alive and in becoming an effective and contributory part of a three-fold family relationship.

In some circles today, parents fill up all their children's leisure time with classes – classes in music, dancing, swimming, gymnastics or judo for example. It seems they want their children to be multiple child prodigies; and they start incredibly early, stationing their unfortunate

---

[*] Leslie Foster, the headmaster of this school, All Saints, pioneered the use of Colour Factor, and wrote the necessary teachers' handbooks.

toddlers in chairs and flashing recognition cards in front of their faces. It is competitiveness run riot. The child is likely to feel oppressed by the responsibility imposed on it to succeed, and quite flattened if it senses that it has failed its parents. The child may gain skills, but with half the day spent in some sort of school and the rest in, or travelling to and from, one of these classes, he has no time to be himself, to choose precisely what he will do or attend to at any moment and become self-reliant and responsible. Nor has he any opportunity to be a spontaneously creative or useful part of a social whole, which he could have, if he were able to play quite spontaneously in the company of a familiar group of children in familiar surroundings, or voluntarily help people with some important and necessary task.

In the United States, there is 'Gymboree' which describes itself as a 'national infant-exercise franchising programme'. In Britain, there is a similar organisation called 'Tumble Tots'. Both are flourishing. The people who have designed these weekly classes for babies and very young children are aware that children learn by doing and that they need much more physical activity than they usually get, and also that they need to spend time in surroundings that have been designed for children's play, 'where parents do not have to say "No" continually'. In an article in *Nursery World*, someone from Tumble Tots is reported to have quoted with approval part of a sentence from *The Self Respecting Child*, 'Toddlers experience a strong desire which will be with them for years, (unless killed of by lack of opportunity to satisfy it) to become acrobatically skilled', and to have added that small children desire to make their bodies do what they want, when they want. *But,* they have only got it *half* right. They and the parents who buy these facilities for their children apparently equate learning with classes – with being taught. They feel it is necessary to *make* the learning happen. Moreover, when the opportunity for learning gymnastic skills is confined to 45 minutes per week, it is understandable that they feel constrained to encourage the children to make the most of the session. The writer of the article on Tumble Tots recalled:

> At Orpington, I watched the two to three year age group as they went through a typical forty-five minute routine. The session began with singing and movement as 14 children, each with a friend or parent, formed a circle to warm up to a taped routine. The level of concentration during this ten-minute period was remarkable – the children were obviously listening and following the leader's instructions carefully. Much of the action depended on timed responses, jumps or shouts in acting out a Jack-in-the-Box for example. Nearly every child had perfect timing and was well-co-ordinated, doing just the right movement at the right time... The equipment is laid out in four or five 'stations' – the children spend seven minutes on each, being guided along and supported by a trainer or parent, before moving to the next piece.

From the rest of the article, it appears that some of the children behave quite spontaneously at times, but, even if the children are not being continually directed and jollied along, the adults taking part evidently outnumber the children and must constitute a somewhat overpowering presence. These classes are better than no opportunity at all to climb, swim, bounce, tumble and slide; how *much* better will depend on the understanding and temperament of the leader ('trainer'). The apparatus provided seems to be good, but its provision presumably depends on the willingness of parents to pay an adequate fee, and they might not be willing if there were no teaching – or at least encouragement and assistance. Moreover the parents are likely to feel greater satisfaction at the end of the session if they have played an active part in it themselves than if they have sat against the wall and watched or chatted.

A sad commentary on modern life was made when the writer describing 'Gymboree' concludes her article:

> It's nice to be able to say 'Yes' to your children and to know you have
> an opportunity to be closer to your child and help him to develop an
> appreciation for exercise (and learning) that can last for a lifetime.

Another effect of the views on child development that are currently predominant in the universities is that the training of the staff of institutions for pre-school education robs them of any faith they may instinctively have in the potential biological wisdom of small children. They find themselves wondering, 'How can we make the children play constructively, talk intelligibly, think logically, feel for others, co-operate, concentrate and learn to follow directions?' instead of, 'How can we create the conditions in which the children may continue the process, begun during their first months, of developing their basic human competence, including the ability to achieve effective relationships with things, physical forces such as gravitation, and mutually enjoyable relationships with other children?'

There is another factor in the situation. As White has pointed out, it is not only children who have a desire to be effective and to exercise a skill they have learned; adults do too. Trained teachers want to teach. If nursery teachers have been taught a variety of ways of keeping children amused, they will want to try them out and to invent more, and will find it difficult to let the children do the inventing. If one's sole occupation is to supervise a group of small children, and one has no consuming interest in the manifestations of biological wisdom, of continuing growth in skill and power, of breadth of interests, of individuality and of the faculty for choice that children display, it is hard to restrain oneself from constantly looming up and intervening between a child and his animate and inanimate environment. It is difficult to let children be.

Little children are so accommodating and polite in what is to them a 'school' situation; they do not often say, 'Buzz off ... you're in my way ... can't you leave me in peace?' And the result is that, unknown and unwept, their power of autonomy is usurped, their biological wisdom and creative individuality are nipped in the bud; a chance to learn to be their own masters, to be responsible for themselves and their environment – for the maintenance of an enjoyable play situation, for example – and to cultivate their power of choice is denied them.

An injection of wisdom from people close to nature

Both developmental psychologists and those engaged in nurturing children can learn a great deal from a study of the way in which the most so-called 'primitive' peoples – the hunter-gatherer (or foraging) peoples – rear their children. Their skill in this field is partly due to the fact that they take it for granted that a small child is a living being which grows because it is it's raison d'être to grow and which, like a flower or a tree, knows how. They also know how to bring up children so that their social impulses tend to prevail over their anti-social impulses. Different peoples have developed different ways of achieving this. But all are loving and indulgent towards babies and little children and provide opportunities for the kind of play that children need and want. Children are also present at adult gatherings and rituals (in which they may play a part traditionally alloted to children), can observe the day-to-day behaviour of adults and older children, and listen to the stories, myths and legends told by the 'elders'. Eleanor Leacock and Richard Lee write in their introduction to *Politics and History in Band Societies*.

> Highly valued by foraging peoples are the qualities of sharing, reciprocity, marrying out, hard work, political equality, sociability and even temper. Contradictions arise when individuals desire to hoard rather than to share, to marry in, to be lazy and freeload, to try to lord it over others, to be sullen and isolate themselves, or to be quick to argue and fight. The ridicule, misfortune or social isolation brought on a person habitually indulging in such behaviour are widespread themes in hunter-gatherer mythology, ritual, child-rearing practice and daily life. The social life of foragers is, in good measure, the continual prevention or working out of potentially disruptive conflicts in accordance with the particular cultural ways of each society. The measure of its success is its record as a viable way of life for by far the greater part of human history.*

The Mbuti Pygmies of the Central African rain forests, of whom I shall have more to say in Chapter 11, knew how to bring up their children to be happy and effective people. Colin Turnbull, who shared their lives for two years and wrote of them in a book† of which Margaret

---

* 1982
† 1961

Meade has said, 'it adds an entirely new dimension to the literature on primitive people,' did not give as much space to babies and children as I could have wished, but he notes that when the hunting band with whom he lived moved to a new camp, which was always close to a stream or river with shallow sandy or pebbly pools, the first thing they did, after building their small houses from branches, brushwood and leaves, was to construct – near the stream – a 'bopi'. This was a playground for the children with swings made of vines, shorter ones for the younger children and one hung from two very tall trees. The children spent their time, tree climbing, splashing and swimming in the river and imitating their elders, playing 'house' – building a house of sticks and leaves, gathering food from the nearby forest and cooking it, and, of course, 'hunting' with tiny bows and arrows. They tell stories in imitation of the adults, repeating what they have heard or making up their own. They also imitate disputes they have witnessed, each taking a role with skilled mimicry. If, on the occasion the children are recalling, the adults talked their way out of the dispute, the children are likely to be content with a straight imitation, but they use their own judgement, and, if they think they could have done better, they will improvise:

> If the adult argument was inept and everyone went to bed that night in a bad temper, then the children try and show that they can do better, and, if they find they cannot, then they revert to ridicule which they play out until they are all rolling on the ground in near-hysterics. That happens to be the way many of the most potentially dangerous and violent disputes are settled in adult life.[*]

Turnbull says that a child has every opportunity to become familiar with and confident within, first his mother's arms, then his parents' 'hearth', then the nearby hearths, then the 'camp' as a whole and finally the forest, with which his people have a mutually sustaining relationship.

Jean Liedloff in *The Continuum Concept*, has described the life of some South American Indians. She was by chance marooned in a Yequana village on the bank of a mountain river in otherwise impenetrable Venezuelan jungle. She returned voluntarily four more times, spending altogether two and a half years with the Yequana people, for, on her return home after her earlier visits, she found it hard to believe that every man, woman and child was as consistently happy as she remembered them to be; they compared so extraordinarily favourably with the people of the North American cities that she knew. They seemed to be uniformly wise in their relationships, their traditional customs, their child-rearing practices and their instinctive knowledge of human psychology.

She found, as anthropologists have found elsewhere, (for example among the Plains Indians of North America) that, in their social and

[*] 1982

economic transactions, they never drove a hard bargain; happy relationships were more important to them than material gain. Their attitude to work was similarly wise: everything necessary was done, but no-one did – or was expected to do – more than he enjoyed doing. She describes illuminating instances of this and also of how they appeared to enjoy difficult and potentially dangerous work. Lengthy and repetitive tasks, such as roofing a house with leaves sewn together, were done co-operatively and made into a party, with plenty of food provided by the owners of the house and, in the evenings, alcoholic drink. Nearly everyone seemed to know, all through life, what was right for him to do in any contingency – what would make for his own happiness, that of his children and the whole village. As Scott Williamson might have put it, their faculty for choice was well developed.

They had had enough contact with industrial civilisation to equip themselves with steel machetes and knives (and they very much appreciated Jean Liedloff's large First Aid box) but most of what they knew of Western civilisation did not attract them. They lived as they had lived for hundreds of generations, hunting in the forest, fishing in the river – a tributary of the Orinoco – and cultivating 'gardens'. The children learned to swim almost as soon as they could walk, and both boys and girls learned astoundingly early to control heavy tree-trunk canoes in the rocky pools of the swiftly flowing river. Liedloff observed that the children were not competitive, very rarely quarrelled and never fought.

The Yequana had strongly individual personalities and were bound by very few rules and taboos. Liedloff attributed their confidence in the rightness and goodness of life and their power to enjoy it to the full to their biological wisdom. She put it that they had not lost their 'continuum sense' – their awareness of and feeling for the needs, tendencies and expectations with which human beings are born and have been born since the human race began. She noticed that they quite effortlessly brought up their children to be truly social adults. Unlike most writers on the lives of 'primitive' peoples, Jean Liedloff observed and described how the babies and small children were treated. Her descriptions are fascinating and 'Western' parents would do well to take note of them.

She observed that their feeling for what is right for themselves as individuals and as human beings was nurtured in them from the beginning of life. They were able to exercise and develop their 'faculty for choice' from birth.

Living with the Yequana made her aware that the new-born baby 'expects' his immediate surroundings and his reception into the world to be similar to those experienced by his forebears. If they are, he feels right.. He is contented and is free to follow his instincts. These lead him to respond to biologically suitable treatment from his family with behaviour that pleases them and encourages them to continue in the same style, for his evolutionarily determined instinct is to behave in a way that elicits good mothering behaviour in people.

So a Yequana baby becomes accustomed to feeling right, and also lovable. For the first month or two of his life, he is held close to his mother's side night and day. Then, until he is ready to enjoy being put on the ground to creep and crawl, he is continually held and dandled, sung and talked to, kissed and hugged by older children and adults alike.

Yequana parents respect their child's biological wisdom. As soon as he becomes capable of learning to creep and crawl, he occupies himself with exploring the world he had until then only known from the viewpoint of some-one's arms, and discovering his own capabilities; he is continuously exercising his faculty for choice and thus developing it. He is careful not to stray far from where his mother is occupied and he goes to her if he needs her. If she has to go any distance, to the river to fetch water for instance, she takes him with her. But at no time does she give him any more or any less assistance than he demands. She never doubts that he will be aware of his needs or that he will exercise his sense of self-preservation and know the limits of his capabilities. And she is right; the Yequana baby continues to do what is right for him – to do what meets his needs – in circumstances which offer a far greater variety of choice than he had as an infant-in-arms. It is no longer always 'involuntary' wisdom that he exercises, but it remains *biological*: it is a response of the whole organism – the whole person – to the whole situation and is exercised in awareness of his needs as a whole.

Liedloff suggests that the way in which we in the 'civilised' West are treated as babies is so contrary to our instinctive expectations that we experience a sense of bitter disappointment. As babies we feel at a loss, and rarely ever recover our sense of what is good and right for us to experience and do. We grow up ignorant both of what is suitable for a human being and of what will make life a misery. We have lost our continuum sense and, therefore, find it difficult to be ideal parents. And yet there are parents who have a relationship of empathy with their babies at the beginning. It is when the babies become toddlers that the conditions of modern life make a parent's task hard indeed. It is difficult to allow children to 'wean' themselves and gradually to widen the sphere of activity in which they can exercise their faculty for choice and, in the process, acquire judgement, confidence and self-esteem. Children can rarely go out to play with the neighbours' children when they feel like it or wander out on their own when mother wants to do some whirlwind spring-cleaning or write or read. An adult and a child are often closeted together far too much, or one child is confined with several adults. Meetings with other children have to be planned in advance and transport arranged.

Forty or fifty years ago it was still possible in some parts of this country (as well as at the PHC) for children to cultivate their power of spontaneous choice and responsibility, their awareness of their surroundings and their wits. Yesterday, I was talking to a window-cleaner I know well and admire. He has always lived on the outskirts of the local small market town. He said, 'On holidays, we used to say to our mother after breakfast, 'See you at tea-time,' and go off to spend the day roaming the nearby lanes and fields and woods, picking blackberries, bird's nesting, collecting conkers and other treasures, and exploring, sometimes for miles... Sometimes we were told off for trespassing, so we avoided that bit next time.' A London-born friend whose feeling of responsibility for others and public spirit I admire, told me that, as children, she and her sister used to walk several miles in a day in search of play-space (from Holborn to Hampstead Heath for example). They had no money, but occasionally managed a short stretch on a bus by the exercise of a little guile.

Today, many parents try to give their children the opportunity to choose, but present the choices in a fairy-tale 'three wishes' manner; there is no constraining reality, no whole situation into which the child must fit himself. For example, they ask a child, 'What would you like to do today? What would you like for dinner? What shall we do tomorrow?' They treat him as they would a guest or someone they particularly wish to placate, constantly trying to ascertain his wishes and desires and themselves adopting the role of selfless attendant. When, as it must be, this course of action is found impossible to maintain, there are tears and rows and terrible feelings of guilt.

In societies like those of the Yequana and Mbuti where adults go about their essential daily tasks and the children are there in the midst of it participating or playing nearby, or further afield, as they wish, children appear to be contented and self-reliant and the parents easy and relaxed. From her observation of the Yequana, Jean Liedloff concluded that a small child 'expects' a strong, busy central figure (or figures) to whom he can be peripheral. He also expects to have the opportunity to be responsible for himself. But to be put into the position of leader is utterly contrary to his expectations. When he is, it confuses and upsets him. Children to whom this happens seem to want more and more attention, help and distraction.

The following is taken from an account of his experiences by an acquaintance of mine who was so impressed by the wisdom contained in *The Continuum Concept* that he decided to practice its implications in his relationship with his six year old stepson, John:

> I started with John more or less at the beginning of our relationship. He would attempt to interrupt whatever I was doing. I was prepared to help him when I decided he could not do whatever it was, but never more than I felt was necessary for him to continue on his own, which was

invariably a lot less than he was asking for. Any other interruption was ignored. If he persisted by grabbing, pushing, or shouting, I moved away to whatever extent was necessary to continue my work, or some other work, but never gave in to the tantrum or reasoned with him angrily or otherwise. On one or two occasions early on, I found myself reasoning with him but soon learnt that this increased his demands, and as I was the one who had to stop these exchanges, it was better not to start. If he showed a respectful interest in what I was doing, I would include him, as long as I could continue. I would have him or my lap, or carried, even if this made my task more difficult, as long as it was not made impossible.

He was never excluded from accompanying me but soon realised that he would simply be with me whilst I was doing whatever I was doing. I enjoy the company of children and, when he was not interrupting, made a point of encouraging physical contact, sharing food, playing, and looked for other opportunities to show that I was interested in his concerns and activities. Concerning food, I never asked him what he wanted, but simply offered some of what I had prepared. If he asked for something different I ignored this. Initially his anti-social behaviour with me increased, and then started to tail off as I remained consistent.

The effect was amazing. After only a week or so, his demands ceased as far as I was concerned, yet he wanted to be with me and accompanied me everywhere. We respected each other's autonomy which produced a spontaneous, free spirited relationship.

Then a woman and her son Tom came to live with them.

Tom's demands and interrupting were much more intensive than John's but after a week or so the same result was achieved. John and Tom sometimes fought. I moved away from them when this occurred, preferably to another room. Their complaints to me about each other were ignored. After a short while, they did not display this behaviour when alone with me.

No Yequana man or woman would dream of carrying a six year old about or having him on his or her lap while working nor would he or she be likely to have to deal with tantrums. But the passage is illustrative of the kind of therapeutic action that may be necessary in our culture.

The intention of many of the people who provide 'counselling' services today is the laudable one of facilitating the patient's own power to decide for himself how to live. They restrict their activity to trying to clarify the problem a person is facing and to bolster his self-confidence. What money and misery might be saved, and what an increase in capability there might be, if people's faculty for choice and for self-reliance were to be allowed to grow without interruption from infancy onwards.

Jean Leidloff was astonished at the extent of the Yequana's respect for a person's autonomy. It seemed that no-one ever attempted to force anyone, adult or child, to do anything against his will. She writes:

Among the Yequana, a person's judgement is thought to be adequate to make any decision he feels motivated to make. The impulse to make a decision is evidence of the ability to do it suitably: small children do *not* make large decisions; they are strongly interested in self-preservation, and, in matters beyond their comprehension, they look to their elders to judge what is best. Leaving the choice to the child from the earliest age keeps his judgement at peak efficiency, either to delegate or to make decisions. Caution asserts itself relative to the responsibility involved, and errors are thus kept to an absolute minimum. A decision taken in this way receives no opposition from the child and therefore works with harmoniousness and pleasure for all.

For the sake of our own health and happiness in the modern world, Liedloff believes it 'is essential to watch for opportunities to reinstate our innate ability to choose what is suitable'. The insights, findings and theories of the Peckham Biologists support this belief.

Chapter 10

The Learning Activity of the Centre Chidren

The Pioneer Health Centre was, as some of it's members began to realise, a place of education. But it was quite definitely not a place where the child is put in the centre and the adults dance attendance on it. A very few only of the member-families would have done this if there had been the opportunity, but there was no opportunity. The children did not want it. And the Biologists and their staff were concerned with the health of families and the growth of every member of the family; their aim was to discover the conditions in which people of all ages can grow and can create around them an ambience that is favourable for growth.

They were interested in the growth of faculties. They observed that babies instinctively do what they need to do in order to learn how to digest food, recognise people, learn the effects of the force of gravity, judge distances, locate sounds, pick up and handle objects, walk, talk and learn how to please the people around them and to obtain from them the reactions they desire to obtain. They saw that a baby is like a sprouting seed whose roots and shoots seek nourishment in the soil, water, air and sunlight, and take in precisely what is needed for the growth and development of the potential characteristics and functions of the plant. He has 'the faculty for choice'.

But the nourishment that the child needs must be present at the right moment. They put it that a baby or a healthy child has an 'appetite' for the particular activities or experiences that will provide the 'nourishment' needed by any one of his faculties at any moment and that he is capable of digesting at that moment.

They realised that opportunities for these experiences and activities must be present or the child's appetite will not be aroused. An interesting experiment which I have described fully in *The Self-Respecting Child* was done on chicks. It was discovered that, although a chicken has an instinct to peck (it pecks it's way out of the shell), it has to learn how to peck grain effectively, and it takes about a day to do so. If kept in the dark and fed by hand for several days after hatching, it becomes incapable of learning to obtain its food in the manner natural to chickens – by pecking.*

Whether or not a baby develops his potential powers and talents depends firstly on his environment, including the way in which he is treated, fed and responded to; and, secondly, on the way he responds to

* Padilla, 1935.

his environment; and this depends on his innate characteristics, including his unique gene make-up, on the nature of his environment and on the nature of his past relationship with his environment. In retrospect, it is impossible to disentangle the threads, to say what has caused a person to be as he is. But one can say that what he is and what he is capable of at any moment is ultimately due to what he himself has felt, pondered on, and, above all, *done* throughout his life to date. Dr Peter Mansfield, a Lincolnshire General Practitioner of Medicine, who is also very actively concerned with people's health and with the means of promoting it in his locality, has put it that 'What we do today we are tomorrow.'

It seems that, if our children are to fulfil their potentiality for growth and development, we must find out what kind of things babies and children in general choose to do and give them the opportunity to do such things. We cannot know what a particular baby or child will choose at any particular moment: only he himself knows what he has an appetite for and what he is capable of digesting at that moment. But we must see that he is free to choose his experiences from among a variety of the kinds that are needed by babies and children if they are to develop fully.

Each child has a different physique and temperament, preferences and priorities, and so it may seem sometimes that for a certain individual it is necessary to provide opportunities for activity of one kind only. I found, however, in my playgroup, that even the most intellectually orientated and physically timid small child would eventually show some interest in 'the slides' (polished hardwood planks, seven feet long with the lower ends resting on the linoleum-covered floor). On one occasion, when we had gone into the garden, I realised that Adam was not with us. I returned to look for him and found him, all alone in the room, walking on hands and feet a few inches up the plank and letting himself slide on his stomach, feet first, on to the floor. He had not dared to do this when other children were present. Some children may seem to be content to sit still and exercise their fingers and eyes only, and, if their surroundings do not make the acquisition of the gross physical co-ordinations easy, may, in later childhood, be clumsy and feeble in certain respects and less able to enjoy many physical and some social activities. Others may take every possible opportunity there is to run, climb, balance, jump and swing and so acquire physical skills and co-ordination of the whole body in spite of an unfacilitating environment. But, when such a child is in the care of people who do not understand this need, the friction and strife engendered may hinder the development of his faculty to relate happily and constructively with other people. Again, some babies may suffer more than others if their human environment fails to give them an understanding and sympathetic response and may, in such a situation, grow up lacking the ability to respond sympathetically to people.

Research into children's learning needs

How do we find what sort of things babies and children need to do in order to develop their potential ability to be fully human – to develop their human faculties and to be rounded, balanced personalities – so that we may give them a suitable environment? Parents and others sometimes know intuitively, or by remembering how they felt as children, or by close and sensitive observation or by the power to see the world through the eyes of a child. At the Centre, we were in a good position to find out how children of all ages will choose to occupy themselves when they are quite free to choose from many alternatives – including doing nothing. We were also in a position to form hypotheses as to the reasons for their choices, what they were learning and what essential faculties and powers they were developing.

The faculty to be aware of which particular experience or activity it is that will at any moment further the development of one's human competence and maturity is like other faculties in that it needs to be used if it is not to decay and be lost. Scott Williamson's biological outlook made him aware of this fact and it was his intention to provide Centre members with the opportunity to exercise the 'faculty for choice' from birth onwards. It soon became clear to him how best to carry out this aim where the adults and the small children in the nurseries were concerned. The school children were a different matter. As has already been told, as soon as the Centre had opened and their parents had joined, the children crowded in. They did not wait for their elders to escort them to the Centre but hurried there as soon as school was over or on holidays at 2pm sharp and ran noisily and excitedly around the building, playing with things that were not intended as playthings and doing minor damage. Scott Williamson refused to segregate them or limit their access to the Centre. In the right circumstances, he believed, healthy children would be responsible children. What were the right circumstances? Of one thing he was sure: one does not encourage health in adults or children by treating them as if they were sick and incapable of exercising responsibility for themselves.

As I described in Chapter 3, the children were allowed to demonstrate that they could be responsible for their own – and others' – safety and enjoyment when they were playing on the climbing ropes, vaulting bucks, wall bars, parallel bars, balancing forms and so on, and that their play involved the exercise and development of precise and accurate physical judgement and co-ordination, as well as other less obvious faculties.

I told also how Lucy Crocker solved the problem of how to allow each child to choose how to occupy himself while he was in the building and to move from one occupation to another with the least fuss and

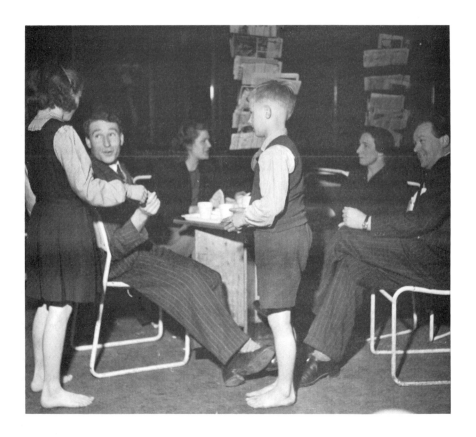

trouble but with the knowledge of a responsible member of the staff. The solution was her 'ticket system'. At first she gave each child that came to her asking for permission to swim or play in the gym a piece of paper on which she had scribbled his name, chosen activity, the date and her initials. Later she had small coloured cards printed with 'Name', 'Activity' and 'Time' followed by spaces for the child to fill in. She carried a bundle around with her – a different colour each day. She also carried a pencil and encouraged the child to fill in the card or, at least, to write his name on it or the nearest he could get to it.

The ticket system proved to serve many important purposes. One of its effects was to accord the children the same privilege as the adult members, who could obtain for three old pence from the cash desk in the Cafeteria a metal counter, which let them through the turnstiles that were situated between the toilets and the men's or women's changing rooms.* A child could do the same with his 'ticket'. From the changing rooms, they could reach either the pool (up a steep flight of concrete steps) or the gym or the learners' pool. It also enabled the staff to treat the children as responsible people. Most important of all, it made freedom of

* After the waar the turnstiles were not restored. Instead a member of staff supervised the area of the learner's pool and the entrance to the gymnasium during the afternoon. The ticket system was used until the end.

choice possible for the children and it provided the Biologists with a record of their choices. Together with the open-view design of the building, it enabled the latter to discover the kinds of play/learning-activity that the children preferred.

This important piece of research into children's needs was made possible by the absence of classes and instructors, for, apart from the spontaneity of choice that this allowed, the children were not influenced in their choices by whether or not they found the instructors attractive people or skilled in teaching; and they were not deterred from trying to learn something for fear of having to commit themselves to attending a class regularly or of finding themselves in a teacher's power and obliged to learn it in his way. They were able to change from one activity to another as their interests changed, without fear of offending anyone.

Another aid to research was the prevailing attitude of Peckham parents at that time. One of the circumstances which enabled the Biologists to be sure that the children were doing what they wanted to do and learning what they chose to learn was that their parents thought of their activity as play and were glad for them to be happily occupied and out of mischief. Today's parents would, I fear, be ambitious for their children's athletic prowess and encourage them to concentrate on some recognised sport or game. They would probably insist on arranging classes for the children so that a teacher could ensure that the children's 'style' was correct from the beginning and could arrange competitions in order to spur the children on. Fifty years ago, parents were less likely to see the future gold medalist or ballerina in their mind's eye. So the children were free to obey their biological instincts; and the Biologists could be sure that the choices were the children's own rather than their parents'.

Since the school age children were free to do what they chose or to do nothing at all, and, in most cases, to go home whenever they liked, the Biologists soon learned which activities were desired and which apparatus, tools and toys were most needed. Lucy Crocker was responsible for deciding what opportunities for activity to provide. Her intuition was sure, but if anything was not used, she withdrew it and, if funds permitted, increased the supply of the more popular equipment.

Our observations, and the records that were made from the used tickets that we collected at the end of the day from the boxes in which the children had left them, showed that as soon as they were allowed to use it – that is when the family had completed their overhauls – the children aged between four and about twelve preferred free-play in the gymnasium to any other activity and usually continued to do so for several weeks. As we watched, it seemed to us that their aim was the acquisition of perfect balance, control and agility – to perfect their power to move precisely as they intended to move in the most exacting circumstances they could devise. It was a delight to watch their rapidly growing skill and grace. Later they would also patronise the swimming pool, or teach themselves to swim in the learners' pool. Having passed the test for the big pool, they played there day after day for months on end, seemingly intent on discovering the possibilities for movement in a new element and the movements in the air that having water below them made possible.

As is common knowledge today, even two year olds love to discover all about the nature of water and what can be done in it as well as with it. The learners' pool at the Centre was emptied every day and filled gradually during the afternoon to a final depth of about three feet. When the water was about nine inches deep, some of the children from the nurseries were taken into it by one of the Curator's 'students'. She found it necessary to be paddling in the pool with the children in order to be immediately at hand to put those who slipped over back on to their feet again: (the heads of children of this age are so heavy in relation to their bodies that once they have inadvertently lost their balance it is difficult for them to get themselves upright again). There was a small platform at one end of the little pool from which three very shallow steps led down into the water, except at the sides where the platform ended in a drop of about a foot (two or three inches above the water level). The 'old hands' would throw themselves into the air from this part of the platform, falling flat with a big splash, stomach first. But it took the children quite a long time to learn how to negotiate the steps and to keep themselves upright in the water. Later they would try sitting down in the water or crawling on hands and knees, until one day they found that the water would hold them up if they stretched out, keeping things under control and moving along by touching the bottom of the pool with their hands. During the time that I was supervising the play two or three of the children learned in the course of their play – no help or instruction was attempted – to trust to their knowledge that the water would support them to succeed in floating on their backs.

At the time, in 1937, I noted:

James Nelson, aged two years and two months is almost master of the situation in water up to one foot. Cannot be quite sure of regaining his feet if he has fallen under, but sits in the water, and also walks on his hands with his legs straight out behind him and his body supported by the water. He loves to watch older (ages three or four) children throw themselves into the water ('dive') from the step – he crows with delight when they do it and obviously longs to do it himself – he never attempts it, and when the water is deeper than usual, he walks extra carefully so as not to fall under.

As I have mentioned, roller skating on the partly covered outdoor

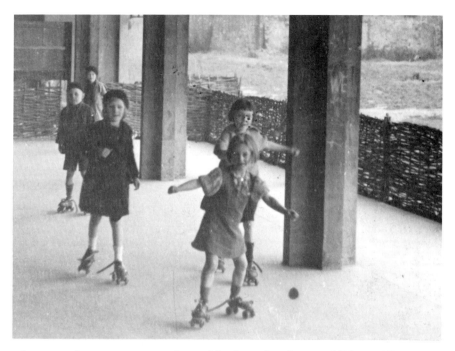

playground was very popular with the school age children. The more proficient liked to play what they called 'shinty' on roller skates with a puck and hockey sticks. The game was similar to ice hockey. The younger ones learned to ride the small bicycles (without stabilisers) and the scooters (with two wheels only, *not* three) that were provided for their use. All these offered them the chance to learn balance and precise control of their limbs. They appeared to welcome the extra complication and hazards afforded by the presence of a number of other children, each moving spontaneously according to his individual purpose. (The shinty equipment was usually issued only in the late afternoon after the younger children had had a chance to skate and ride bikes and scooters.)

Having spent several weeks or months satisfying these apparently basic and essential needs, most of the children became interested also in activities that require and promote more specialised or finer co-ordinations or a more abstract form of judgement such as draughts or chess, drawing, sewing, reading, writing, using an old typewriter, table tennis, billiards, badminton, diving or ballroom dancing.

Throughout, it seemed to us, the children were engrossed in occupations that would promote the development of their faculties – physical, intellectual and social. Scott Williamson said they were engaged in the process of 'facultisation'. He remarked that one should not expect children to welcome the opportunity to acquire culture until they have achieved a degree of facultisation that satisfies them.

Facultisation – sensory-motor

It seemed to be the case that many of the children, at the time their families joined the Centre, felt themselves to be short of opportunities for developing their faculty for precise, swift, economic and appropriate movements of the body as a whole – for what is most accurately described as 'general sensory-motor judgement'.

Books on children very rarely, if ever, describe the activity of toddlers who are engaged in the process of acquiring general sensory-motor judgment, learning the niceties of balance and how to respond advantageously to the gravitational pull with every muscle, because almost no-one has thought it worth noticing. The biologist, Milicent Shinn, is an exception. In the detailed diary she kept of the behaviour of her niece Ruth, she observes:

> During all this period [from the age of around 15 months] a noticeable trait was the child's interest in doing something novel with her body, apparently in mere curiosity and sense of power. In the sixty-first week she found she could walk with her head thrown back, looking at the ceiling, and practised it for a long time. In the sixty-fifth week she walked about in her father's slippers, lifting her encumbered feet skilfully. At sixteen months she hit upon the feat of walking backwards and practised it all day, much interested and amused. In the seventieth week, her great joy, when indoors, was a shallow box, some two and a half inches high, upon which she would stand, stepping on and off with endless pleasure.*

Ruth was developing her sensory-motor judgement and the control of and co-ordination of the movements of her limbs and body as a whole. In *The Self-Respecting Child*, I have quoted more from Milicent Shinn's book, because Ruth's behaviour is typical of the spontaneous activity of children of this age. They are exercising and developing their muscles, motor nerves, senses of sight and balance and the network of nerves and sense organs known as the proprioceptor system. Obviously a child cannot learn to step on and off a box with precision and perfect balance until he has acquired enough co-ordination and judgement to be able to walk forwards and to bend and straighten his knees without overbalancing. In other words, he must have already acquired a certain amount of general sensory-motor judgement. Then, on this existing sensory-motor body-of-knowledge, he grows – through his activity – a new 'limb', the knowledge of how to step on to and off a box of a certain size.

There is a further reason for the large amount of time that children need to spend learning general sensory-motor judgment. It is that they grow, and therefore need to ensure that their knowledge keeps pace with the gradual alteration in their stature and proportions, and the increase in

* 1909

and distribution of their weight. It is not only that the child's muscles need to be stronger because of the increasing weight and length of his limbs, but also that the activity of all the parts of the body in the performance of any particular movement needs to be very slightly different week by week as the child grows. The manner in which gravity affects the body during any particular movement changes with the change in the proportions, size and weight of the body; and the child's directing sensory-motor intelligence has to be kept up to date with this changing data. The child that grows fast needs to spend more time doing this than the stocky or lightly-built, small-boned type, if he is to achieve the same amount of general sensory-motor co-ordination and judgement.*

It is fair to guess that the acquisition of general sensory-motor judgement and co-ordination gives a child a satisfying feeling of potential effectiveness; he feels capable of doing precisely what he intends to do (at least after a little practice) in the physical field. This gives him a feeling of security, just as confidence in his ability to deal with eventualities of all kinds, and to enjoy life, will give him a sense of security.

If a physically well co-ordinated child wishes to become expert in any particular sport, he will be able to do so the more quickly and easily. Specialist training is productive of skill in proportion to the degree of general sensory-motor judgement and co-ordination that the child already possesses and is still acquiring through spontaneous play in suitable surroundings.

Coaching and training have their uses. If a child is ambitious, he may want to undergo a period of training under instruction at some time or other; but training can never be an effective substitute for the spontaneous, self-selected and self-initiated practice that occurs during play. Judgement in any field can only be acquired through the exercise of judgement. A child who performs prescribed exercises will learn how to perform those exercises more or less well and may become more supple and muscularly strong but little more. The speed and ease with which he is able to learn how to perform different exercises will not be increased. Training does not enable the child's body of general sensory-motor knowledge to grow as does spontaneously self-chosen play. It is as if the child that is being trained in a particular skill is suffering forced feeding with one type of food only, while the child playing in an appropriate environment is taking exactly what he needs, at the particular moment in time, for growth; he is growing a sturdy, bushy tree of knowledge which is capable of putting out a new shoot in any direction at any moment.

It is interesting to compare these findings from the Peckham experiment with Piaget's observations on the experimental training of babies detailed in Chapter 9.

An interesting observation of the effects of training was made by the Peckham Biologists (1943):

* See *The Self-Respecting Child*, Chapter 7

We had in the Centre one interesting example of the inhibiting effect that training may induce. Some of the children who spent a good deal of time diving and who were deemed very promising material, were enthusiastically and methodically taught by a professional – a trainer of competitors for the Olympic Games. He was an extremely good teacher and evidently an inspiring one, as the children rushed to learn with him. But what happened to those whose enthusiasm carried them through a strenuous course? As soon as their teacher stopped coming, they stopped diving, and some of them never took it up or dived again with any enthusiasm.

Functional efficiency has to be acquired in infancy and childhood. As the existing social and educational systems tend progressively to deprive children at an increasingly young age of their biological inheritance, it is no wonder that training is more and more coming to be considered a necessity for youth – though not, of course, by its advocates recognised as therapy.

Easy, smooth, graceful and precise movement may be partly the reflection of temperament and attitude to life, but it is also the effect of the possession of general sensory-motor judgment. In fact, without the latter, feeling cannot be expressed adequately. Therefore ease and grace of movement is not by any means entirely a gift from heaven. It cannot be taught, but it must be learned.

Appetitive phases

The following are illustrations of the selectivity of young children's appetites for learning, and of the lengths to which they will go in order to satisfy their desire for a certain skill. The first I found among the regrettably infrequent notes that I made during the time I was working at the Centre:

> January 22nd. Brian O [aged just four] was away from school owing to a cold – asked for skates, insisted on keeping them on for three hours. The next day he had them on for 4 hours and the same every day for a week. By the end of the week he could skate fast and well and turn corners with skill.
>
> Brian was a bit anti-social in the nursery and uncontrolled in his behaviour. Now that he goes to school, comes to the Centre on his own and goes when and where he likes, he is a responsible person. No-one bothers about him and he bothers no-one else. There was a very short period at first when he was up to mischief.

Of many instances in my playgroup, I remember particularly the example of Kathy. At the age of three and a half, Kathy was determined to ride a bicycle. I had, with difficulty, obtained some very small scooters with only a single wheel at the back instead of two, and I had succeeded in finding two second-hand small bicycles without stabilisers or any frills such as mudguards, so that they were as tough and light as possible, but had had to have the frames cut down so that the saddle was low enough for a small three year old to reach the ground with both feet simultaneously. Our four elder children had all learned to ride before they were five on a conventional 'fairy cycle', again with no stabilisers, but at four they were already long-legged and they had the advantage of being able to use the level pavement outside our house which was in a quiet street. The playgroup children had to make do with our back garden which was sloping except for a small rough lawn with steeply downward sloping banks on three sides and occupied by a low and spreading apple tree (ideal for climbing) and other pieces of climbing apparatus and toys. Most of the children progressed no further than learning the art of scooting down the sloping paths, astride the seat, learning to balance and steer while holding their legs out beyond the whirring pedals of the little fixed-wheel bikes. But Kathy was determined to ride properly. She never requested help, but whenever the weather permitted play out of doors, she went straight for a bicycle, waiting for one to be free if necessary, keeping her eyes fixed on them and whoever was using them and never allowing herself to be distracted by anyone or any other activity. Taking the bike on to the level part of the lawn, she would try and try again, until one day she had achieved the co-ordinations necessary for pedalling while balancing and steering all without help or advice.

At the Centre, it was observed that when a child had worked – sometimes every day for weeks – at mastering a particular skill, he would revel for a while in his newly acquired power and then move on to the mastery of something else, even if it meant changing his play-fellows. It appeared that between the age of five and about eleven, (apart from a few inseparable pairs, often two brothers or sisters close together in age) choice of activity was more important to the children than choice of companions.

I think we were justified in believing that, in choosing to spend so much time in the acquisition of general sensory-motor judgment, the children of the members of the PHC were satisfying their own instinctive needs rather than emulating their elders. There was as yet (before the war) very little television and, although in the mid thirties many governments were beginning to foster the ideal of physical fitness, it had not in 1936 yet taken hold in Peckham. So I think that the children must have been motivated entirely by their instincts – by the primitive human within – what Laurens van der Post calls the 'first man', which, he says, 'it is important for human survival and happiness that we deliberately recover'.

In most parts of the modern world, it is possible to reach maturity and successfully rear a family, and to reach positions regarded as the highest in the land without having acquired the ability to leap over a fence without catching one's foot, cross a river by means of a narrow tree trunk or pull oneself on to the bough of a tree or a rocky ledge above one's head, whereas abilities such as these were necessary for *survival* for most of the time that humans have been on the Earth. Perhaps that is why children usually rejoice in their acquisition and adults often see no point in it. But some people do admit that the possession of such abilities can add to a young person's confidence, self-respect and joy in living.

It is of course not true that all children seek to obtain general sensory-motor judgement throughout their childhood. Most do at the toddler stage, but some soon lose confidence in their ability to acquire it, just as some lose confidence in their ability for intellectual attainment. But it is reasonable to suppose that, if children can find – and take – plenty of opportunities to develop agility and balance while their centre of gravity is still close to the ground and before they have put on much weight, they are likely to continue to respond to opportunities to develop these powers as they grow taller and heavier. If, on the other hand, they fail to acquire general sensory-motor judgment, control and co-ordination early, there may come a time when the gap in the sequence of development becomes unbridgeable. With application, such individuals may be able to make up for lost time to some extent when they have stopped growing, but they are likely to have suffered throughout their childhood and youth from a sense of inadequacy and an inhibiting fear of finding themselves unequal to the challenges they may encounter at any time.

Facultisation – social

It was less obvious that the children were developing the faculty for harmonious and creative relationships with other children. I realised that the Centre children were doing this when later I recalled their behaviour after I had watched the children in my pre-school playgroup acquiring competence in personal relationships, and in creating easy and happy play situations.

In a 'free-choice playgroup', no-one instructs the children to play with each other. If a child wants the co-operation of others in his play, he must take their feelings and desires into account to some extent or he will not retain their company; they will leave him and his game for one of the many other occupations that are available. So, unless a child wants to play solo all the time, he will soon begin to learn the art of co-operation and give-and-take; he will exercise and develop his potential ability to be aware of others' feelings and begin to learn about human nature in its infinite variety.

The following is an extract from *The Self-Respecting Child*. It illustrates the need children have to learn about people and situations through their senses. At the age of two or three, words mean little. At this age, children can only learn about things and other people and themselves through physical and emotional experience and by experimenting. It also illustrates the satisfaction and joy it gives little children to acquire both sensory-motor and social skills and to gain, on their own initiative, the ability to respond effectively to the challenges of their environment.

Recently a little boy of Ghanaian parentage has joined our group. He is two years and three months old, very strong and active, intelligent, curious, playful and determined. He is less well acquainted with toys than most of the other children were when they joined the group, and, apart from exploring the house and garden and pushing and pulling everything that it appears to him to be safe to push and pull and that responds interestingly to being pushed and pulled, he likes to open and shut doors and to use objects that are familiar to him, such as a dustpan and brush – which he wields effectively – and scissors, for his mother makes her own clothes. Apparently it gives him confidence, in this new and very strange environment, to exercise the skills in which he is already proficient.

During his first week or two in the group, he was hardly still for a moment. He would rattle small objects such as beads in their box and then suddenly turn the box upside down – but he would sometimes help to pick them up again. He would seize a paint-brush, dab at the paper, then at his hand, his shoes, the wall or the floor, or he would push the easel over. (Our easels invite a push because they consist simply of two pieces of hardboard joined together at the top and standing in a tray.) He would suddenly throw things – often over his shoulder without watching where they went; or he would throw himself to the floor and roll about. But he liked to sit in the 'Home Corner' alone or with another child – sometimes for several minutes – 'pouring' from the teapot and 'drinking' from a cup.

He is cautious in his use of the slides and the climbing frame. For the first two weeks he used them rarely and did not trust himself to go more than about a foot from the ground. During the third and fourth weeks he climbed higher but very carefully and prudently. He strode away muttering to himself when he caught sight of the towering figure of my son with his long blond hair, but is not in the least deferential towards adults who have proved themselves to be friendly.

On arrival in the group, he was obviously completely ignorant of other children. As his mother said, 'He only knows Daddy and me.' His behaviour towards them, if they were the same size or smaller than himself, was similar to his behaviour towards inanimate objects; he investigated them and experimented on them in an impulsive and muscular way, including pinching, pulling and occasionally biting. We had to watch him constantly during the first few days, and sometimes to advise the victims to hit back. He was visibly surprised if they did so, and would pause a moment, apparently in thought, before turning to explore some other part of his surroundings. After four weeks in the group he is both more cautious and more confident in his approach to the children.

He is, in fact, learning incredibly quickly how to enjoy the playgroup, and the company of the other children. He has been asked not to throw or upset things, and in order to make our meaning clear to him we have sometimes taken things away from him. Now he will remain at one occupation for quite a few minutes and enjoys using the pegboard pegs for their intended purpose instead of throwing them around the room. He realizes that the paper on the easel is meant for painting on, although he cannot always resist the temptation to daub other things.

One day, after he had been in the playgroup for about a week, two or three of the children had made some 'swords' out of plastic 'meccano' – very pliable and wobbly weapons – and they were playing at clashing their 'swords' together. Kuase somehow got hold of one for a moment and succeeded in joining in the game. This pleased him so much that, grinning broadly, he ran and literally leapt on to the rocking horse – which up to then he had not had the courage to use – and then proceeded to rock himself carefully and attentively for a minute or two.

His mother appears to find him a great source of amusement, which is fortunate since his curiosity, determination and energy might otherwise have caused her nerves to snap in the constricted conditions of her home. Having watched his debut in the playgroup she asked the supervisor one day, 'Do you think he is a little bit daft?', a question which brought the strongest of sincere denials. Later she told us that, since he has been coming to the playgroup, he has been appreciably more gentle towards herself and more amenable than he was before.

I have described Kuase's behaviour for two reasons. It was easy to follow the processes that were going on in him because he acted so spontaneously and expressed his feelings so uninhibitedly in movement and facial expression. Secondly, he was, at the time he joined the group, physically strong and mature for his age and also potentially very capable; therefore his behaviour demonstrated very clearly the extent of his ignorance of the creatures, objects and situations that he found in the playgroup when he joined it, and also the speed at which he was learning judgment of every kind.

However, the acquisition of social judgment is only possible – even in a playgroup or nursery school – when supervisors and organizers are aware of the importance of freedom. If they are not, they may unwittingly make it very difficult for the children to develop this faculty.

It so often happens that a child joining a playgroup or nursery – both of which, I am sorry to say, are nowadays usually referred to as 'play-school' – is told that he is a big boy now and is going to school. He watches to see what behaviour is expected of him in this new situation. If he finds that 'school' is a place where you do what teacher wants, he may be content to be told what to do and how to do it. He puts up with it, if 'teacher' cuts short his train of thought, his appreciation of the experience of his senses and feelings or his close observation of the doings of the other children with, 'Now we'll do music [or] cooking,' or, 'Come and see what Joan has done. She has put a car on one side of the balance and a truck on the other and the truck is heavier than the car. Look, it is as heavy as two cars'; or, just when he is about to share an important discovery he has made with his friend Joe, or just when the slide is unoccupied and he has summoned up the courage to go down it for the first time, or just as he has decided on the course of action that is most likely for successful participation in Jill's game of Mothers and Fathers, the adult says, 'What would you like to do Jimmy? What about painting? No? Sand? No? Well come and listen to a story.' After a bit he finds it is not worth his while to take the trouble to exercise his powers of awareness, sensibility, discrimination, choice or will. He may become inwardly passive and empty although apparently busy and happy enough. He may become conditioned to being jollied along and entertained. Or he may find it best to appear to be busy in order to avoid being pounced upon and made to decide 'what he would like to do'.

In the Centre nursery, this sort of thing never happened, and, after they had grown out of the nursery, the children were able to go on to practise both sensory-motor and social judgement – and also responsibility – in the wider environment of the Centre building as a whole.

During the period from 1936 to 1939, some primary schools in Peckham took children from the age of three and a half (probably owing to a recent lowering of the birth rate). Therefore, some of the members' children began to attend school soon after they had reached that age. Because they were at school and no longer attending the Centre nursery, they were, if their parents allowed it, promoted to the freedom of the whole building. The four year old Brian O, mentioned above, was one of these. Both his home and his school were quite near the Centre, and his parents allowed him to go to there on his own. He had a sister about four years older than himself who used the Centre almost every day, and this may have given them and him confidence in his safety, although I do not remember her as a mothering type.

I cannot recall any other specific individuals as young as Brian coming in and out on their own, but there must have been a number of very young children that were keen to acquire the physical skills being demonstrated by older children, because I remember that no bicycles and roller skates small enough to fit these tots were obtainable in this country, and that the management were forced to go to France for one and the USA for the other.

The 'ticket system' combined with the open-view design of the building facilitated the extension of a most unusual degree of freedom to these small children, for by these means the Curator was able to be aware of the doings and whereabouts of the children, only restricting their movements by refusing them permission if necessary to a particular activity at a particular time. For example, she reserved the gymnasium for the younger or less experienced children during the first half of the afternoon (from 4pm to 5pm). The Curator and the child were able to meet in mutually advantageous circumstances and to make recurrent contact and acquaintance. Moreover, since the children had to find the Curator wherever she might be in the building, probably anywhere except in her 'office', and often in conversation with adult members, they found themselves moving about among the adults and the older children and could watch what was going on. It gave them the opportunity to indulge the natural curiosity most children feel concerning the adult world and what makes adults tick. They could learn by the same means they had used from birth – by watching. And the adults and older children served quite unconsciously as models for behaviour. The children, by keeping quiet and their eyes and ears open, were able to pick up some useful social skills as they went looking for the enabling ticket. As I have noted elsewhere, the presence of the adults was a safeguard to them in their immaturity. It also gave them the opportunity to see what new ideas for activity the activities engaged in by the adults and older children might suggest to them. As I noted of Brian O, it sometimes happened that children who had chafed a little at being confined to the nursery where the opportunities for physical activity may not have been – to them – sufficiently consistently challenging, responded to greater freedom and opportunity with increased maturity of behaviour, after a very short period of wildness.

As I have already noted, the children between the age of five and about twelve followed their appetite for sensory-motor skills where it led them. What they did was more important to them than who they did it with. But, as adolescence approached, we noticed a change. Groups formed. We noticed certain children taking great trouble to meet each other at pre-arranged times in order to swim or play some game together. We were aware of this because at about six in the evening when we were having our supper break, a boy or girl would come for a ticket and then wait about until a small group had collected with their tickets when they would go off all together. This change to a liking to do things in a particular group was heralded at the age of about eleven by the momentary emergence of small gangs of one sex that formed, it appeared, for the purpose of teasing or chasing – or being chased by – a gang of the opposite sex. The seizure of someone's cap or school hat (this was the age of ubiquitous hat or cap wearing) was often the instigatory action.

There was a group of boys who frequented the 'wireless room' and, at one time, a group of 12 to 14 year olds that centred round a boy of about 16 who had a passion for making up plays and 'producing' them. This group used the theatre stage for a few weeks or perhaps months, in the interval between the afternoon and the evening badminton or the dramatic society or Concert Party rehearsals. Elvet Chapman who remembered being one of this group fifty years ago told me:

The plays had Frankenstein themes. We never played to an audience. Once or twice some adults came in and watched for a bit. This boy loved creating and making up things and telling us what to do and say, and we enjoyed it... There was a machine that made a noise like the wind... I don't remember whether there were any girls in the group or not.

There was a long-lasting group of boys and girls whose special interest was badminton. I remember they would come to the Centre about six o'clock and borrow the shuttlecock and racquets that were loaned to the children. Lately, I talked to Adge Elven who told me he was a member of this group throughout its existence. He recalls with pleasure his experiences at the time, nearly fifty years ago. He clearly remembers most of the individuals who shared his enthusiasm for badminton at this time; with some he made firm friendships that lasted for many years after the Centre had closed. He told me how the keenest of the boys and girls would sit and watch the adults playing and, when they stopped for a half-time break, would themselves take possession of the court, and that these 12 to 15 year olds produced a team that regularly beat the adults' third team and, on one memorable occasion, their second team. He told me that the preference of a nucleus of the group for badminton continued until the Centre closed at the outbreak of war, although they also enjoyed other activities, played in the gym and swam together – or, rather, played in the swimming pool. He remembered, incidentally, that the sports coach at his school had told him that he would never make a really good swimmer and would be better to concentrate on cricket and football, but to go swimming once a week with his class.

> It was about that time [Adge said] that I joined the Centre. I swam every evening, or, rather, I played in the pool with my friends and dived a lot, but we only skylarked... I suppose I became water-worthy. One day, at school, the swimming coach brought the school team into our class and asked the master to pick out some boys to swim against the team to give them some practice. I beat my chap by a yard, so I was in the team there and then.

This, Adge felt, was an example of the advantages of 'playing' over conventional training. He recalled that he and some of his friends had, for a period, a daily routine: they played badminton for about an hour, then played in the gym for about half an hour and then jumped into the pool when the eight o'clock bell went. Swimming for only half an hour at a time was a rule, Adge said, 'Miss Crocker enforced it. She was quite a dragon to us, but we respected her – she was fair, that's very important with children.' In the summer holidays, as our records showed, some children would swim twice a day.

Some of this informal association of boys and girls were less avid badminton players than Adge, and one got the impression that they were motivated more by the desire to get to know a number of individuals well, to learn about others and themselves and to practise the art of interacting happily and effectively with others of their age. Indeed, it seemed to us likely that all these young people were motivated to some extent by this desire. Perhaps, like the children in the gym and the nursery and in my playgroup, they were enjoying the opportunity to learn the art of being themselves and at the same time contributory parts of a harmonious social whole – the art of being me and also us.

At the Centre, there was plenty of opportunity for continuity of association with individuals of one's choice. In order to meet a person frequently, teenagers had no need to go in for 'dating' and thus get involved in tight and emotionally fraught one-to-one relationships, before they felt capable of coping with them. There was less danger of getting caught in a habit-forming relationship, of making a habit of going around with a person whom one had not at all carefully chosen in the first place.

Moreover, young people could engage in occupations that require companions and the acquisition of social skills, and become acquainted with a variety of individuals without being obliged to tie themselves down to a particular leisure-time pursuit by joining, for example, a club for badminton only or enrolling in a dancing class. They could easily move from one group to another or stay on the fringe of several. The Centre was a place with the accessibility of a village green but also offering shelter, light and warmth.

Towards the end of the pre-war period, it became evident that many of the members' children were making smooth and steady progress into adulthood. I remember some, in their teens when war broke out, whose families re-joined immediately it was over and who, as young adults, made a memorable contribution to the life of the post-war Centre.

Not all the members' children made the very varied use of the Centre that I have described. There were a few particularly shy and retiring ones, and a few who preferred the books and bits of handicraft, available in Lucy Crocker's cabinets in the 'office' off the cafeteria, to the more vigorous activities.

There were some – usually 'only' – children who were what Dr Pearse called 'skirt-bound'. They had remained dependent on their mother's presence long after it was necessary. In some cases, if the children were young enough and the mother realised what they were missing, she was able to take advantage of the opportunities that membership of the Centre offered to encourage them to be more independent, just as animals push their young away at a certain stage to fend for themselves. But some mothers had themselves become dependent on the dependency of the child. Mother and child had become parasitic on each other to such an extent that neither could extricate herself and stand on her own feet, or seek nourishment elsewhere and grow. It was guessed that this situation had sometimes caused a family to give up its membership. Their inability to enjoy the Centre frightened them. I remember Lucy Crocker remarking that the children whose mothers had been in the habit of allowing them out to play in the streets (not an irresponsible action in those days) were better off than those who were more carefully brought up and kept constantly under the parent's eye.

The growth of self-esteem

The following is from the notes I made in 1936:

> The children are often shy and self-consciously good at first. After a week or two some get wild and take advantage of the freedom of the place for a short while. They then soon settle down to use it sensibly.

The building, with its simple open-plan design and the continual movement of people around it, always contained people of various ages. At no time did it only contain children. From 2pm when it opened there were always some shift or night workers coming in for a swim or a game of billiards as well as some of the mothers of young children who spent much of their leisure there, and the example of their relaxed and civilised behaviour must have had its effect on the children. But the children were responsible for themselves: the adults were not there in order to control the children; they were there for exactly the same purposes as the children – to amuse and entertain themselves and to grow. Another cause of the maturity of demeanour displayed by the children was surely that they were never bored. They never had to stand kicking their heels in a queue: if their first choice of activity was by chance fully booked, there were always others on which to spend a short time while waiting. When they had had enough for that day of what the Centre offered, they went home. In those days in Peckham, mothers of children of school age were rarely in paid employment outside the home, so the children were not shut out of the house; they were not obliged to remain in the Centre for lack of somewhere else to go. Moreover, play in the streets was more possible then than it is now. The children were their own masters, free to come and go. Also, within the Centre, they were free at any time to remove themselves from the open forum they shared with the adults to the kind of environment that only children can appreciate and enjoy, such as that which they created for themselves in the gymnasium and outdoor playground. They were free to choose.

Pearse and Crocker write (1943):

> ... let us make no mistake about it, the child has no wish to be relegated to a world of its own. The world of its parents, of the grown-ups, is a

place of mystery and enticement to it and, as it grows, it longs to share in it more and more.

This is, I think, still true in spite of the precocious sophistication caused by television. At least, it is true of young children; older ones are inclined to look forward only as far as entry to the adolescent world, beyond which their ambitions do not extend. Perhaps this is because they are aware that their parents' generation have allowed the adolescent to be the trend-setter and may therefore seem to be on the decline themselves, to be already has-beens.

Certainly, there was no doubt at all that the Centre children enjoyed being in the adult world without wanting to play a central part in it. The table games, billiard cues, table tennis bats etc. available for the children's use were kept in the outer section of the Curator's 'office', off the Cafeteria. The children helped themselves after obtaining a ticket which they deposited in lieu. Therefore there was a constant coming and going of children in and around the part of the building where adults chose most often to sit. If there were spaces free at the tables in the Cafeteria, the children would sit down with their Ludo or draughts, jigsaw puzzles or homework right among their seniors. They were not self-consciously quiet or on their best behaviour; they certainly did not whisper in corners, but neither were they intentionally obtrusive, trying to draw attention to themselves, self-consciously crowding, giggling and 'showing off'.

Although many things contributed to the rapid development of the children's astonishingly mature and responsible behaviour, I judge that the basic underlying cause was the fact that they had been able to satisfy their appetite for the kind of mental and physical activity that is dear to the hearts of children, and not only a general appetite but the precise and particular need of the moment. I believe that most of the Centre children enjoyed the comfortable feeling of being well-nourished functionally, of being competent and effective in ways that were important to them, I think that this feeling was behind the serenity and purposefulness of the children and their friendly straight-forward manner that was remarked upon by staff, members and visitors alike. With very few exceptions, they did not seem to be subject to destructive or anti-social impulses. If they had felt such impulses, they would have had a strongly felt motive for controlling them: one does not kill the goose that lays the golden eggs. It was evident that the Centre provided them with the opportunity to spend every minute doing what they wanted above all else to do. This was to exercise and develop their potential human faculties – the faculties that make for human competence and maturity. After it had been made possible for children of all ages to grow smoothly in this way, it was only very rarely that anyone had a complaint to make about the behaviour of a child. Indeed, before long, people were finding that the completely unorganised presence of the children throughout the building made a pleasant, interesting and amusing addition to the society of the Centre. The adults did not merely accept the presence of the children; they enjoyed having them around, both their own and other people's. This, in turn, increased the self-esteem of the children and their respect for the adults.

I think it is insufficiently understood that children have as great a need to feel effective as to feel lovable. It is necessary to their self-respect to feel confidence in their growing powers. At every stage in their growth, they seek evidence of their ability to be effective and skilled and are happy when they find it. All observant parents must notice this and yet it is not generally accepted as a fact. Because people do not recognise the existence of this universal need, the environment of small children may not be conducive to self-respect, self-confidence and joy. Indeed it can happen that a child is so seriously deprived of these feelings that he becomes ill; he may develop a form of childhood schizophrenia. Modern foodstuffs may be a contributory cause, as they are of much ill-health, but a child who is particularly sensitive to a feeling of powerlessness may be especially at risk if he is in the care of people who do not allow him to have what he feels is an effective relationship with them or with his physical surroundings, or if they expect him to behave and develop in ways that are impossible for him. For fear of further repulse or failure and humiliation, he may retreat into himself, shrink from contact with people and turn his back on such opportunities as there are for experience and action. And so it comes about that he is deprived of the chance to build the foundations of a person – to become fully human.

In *The Empty Fortress*, Bruno Bettelheim describes extreme cases of this kind that were brought to him for treatment, and what he and his dedicated staff were able to do for them at the Orthogenic School in the University of Chicago*.

Bettelheim says:

> What humanises the infant is not being fed, changed or picked up when he feels the need for it... It is rather the experience that *his* crying for food brings about *his* satiation by others according to *his* timing that makes it a socialising and humanising experience. It is that *his* smile, when it is an invitation to play, results in being played with.†

Virginia Axline describes, in an unforgettable little book, *Dibs in Search of Self*, how she helped an exceptionally intelligent little boy, (he was later to have an IQ of 168) who, at the age of five, was rapidly reverting to infancy – but a sullen and viciously aggressive one – and was likely to become classified as mentally deficient. As a psychotherapist, she was called in to treat him, and she brought him back to health

* See *The Self-Respecting Child* for a short account of this
† 1967

and happiness during a series of weekly sessions in a therapeutic playroom. There he played, without any lead from her, gradually talking more and more about what he was doing. She showed that she was taking a respectful interest in what he did and said, often by repeating his statements but without making any even remotely critical or 'educative' comments or any suggestions as to what he might do or play with. She happened to meet him in the street two and a half years after the nine months or so of therapy had ended and he said:

> 'I know you. You are the lady of the wonderful playroom... I remember how you played with me.' 'What did we play, Dibs?' 'Everything I did, you did. Everything I said, you said.'

The perspicacious Swiss Professor of Natural History, Karl Groos, writing at the turn of the century,* observed that children manifest 'joy in being a cause'; they have a healthy appetite for power.

There was a mother who always arrived at my playgroup holding her four year old tightly by the hand, although they lived literally just around the corner. I called on her one day, and during my visit, which was in the afternoon, the little boy spent a lot of time turning the light on and off, while closely observing the effect on us. I do not think he was behaving like this in order to get attention; he received plenty – indeed, too much – *unsolicited* attention from his mother. Rather, because he knew his mother would not smack or lecture him in front of a visitor, he seized a rare opportunity to be effective and to feel powerful.

Sometimes a child may channel his desire to be effective into learning how to predict his parents' reactions to events and become extremely skilled at 'bending them around his little finger'. It may be that the child has insufficient opportunity to become skilled in other fields of activity or it may be that he (or perhaps more often she) prefers the skill of manipulating other people to other skills. He may test his skill by being as contrary as he dares, judging just how far it is politic to go.

At the Centre no instance of bullying was ever observed by any member of staff. There appeared also to be no 'daring' of each other by the children during their play. I can think of three possible reasons for this absence of aggressive power seeking. Firstly, they had no need to repel boredom by teasing, competing, fighting, establishing dominance or other potentially anti-social and dangerous activities. Secondly, each child was aware that he, together with the other children, was responsible for the preservation of the play-situation that he valued so highly; and thirdly, having acquired considerable power over themselves and over physical forces and things, they had little desire for power over other people, and felt no compulsion to boost their self-esteem by obtaining it.

Could vandalism and bullying be caused by a long-endured and unsatisfied hunger to feel effective, I wonder; could they be compensatory activi-

* 1901

ties, undertaken, in order to bolster self-esteem, by doing something – anything – that makes one feel powerful or that impresses 'the gang'?

The growth of responsibility

Perhaps one of the reasons why there is, it seems, less irresponsible and anti-social behaviour among the young in 'primitive' societies is that there the children can, from an early age, spend all the time they wish in play that gives them exquisite physical co-ordination and agility as well as social skill; they can watch adults and older children at work and at play; they can attend most social occasions and, in their play, imitate what they have seen and heard and thus gradually acquire the knowledge and skills that make them effective hunters, gatherers and preparers of food, singers, dancers and story-tellers. Moreover they can often feel that they are useful members of the family or tribe by imitating the adults work and by taking on small jobs that are within their capabilities and that it is evident to them are necessary for the welfare of the group. To a lesser extent, the Centre children had opportunities to feel satisfyingly effective and at home in the world.

The Biologists were surprised at the Centre children's complete lack of competitiveness. Below the age of 13 or 14 they never organised competitions or races among themselves or asked anyone to do so for them. They seemed to have no desire to prove that they could do better than the next child or to compare their skill with that of others. Sometimes they played games that entailed winning or losing and to that extent enjoyed competition with others but it was evident that their pleasure lay mainly in the acquisition of a skill to their own satisfaction or in solving a problem or meeting a challenge that they had chosen for themselves.

The phrase 'meeting a challenge' may give a false picture, for the children did not give the impression of being engaged in struggles with themselves or anything else; they seemed to be doing only what came easily to them. Yet they were far from being lax or lackadaisical. It was noted that on a Saturday afternoon many of them were engaged in one strenuous activity after another for three or four hours with hardly a break. In spite of this expenditure of energy, they showed no signs of fatigue such as a lack of restraint or loss of concentration that may lead to faulty judgment and accidents. Perhaps they did not get tired because they were satisfying their present appetite for skill and were not greedily trying to swallow what they were at the time incapable of digesting; they were not pushing themselves to attain a standard set by someone else, nor were they trying to 'beat' the other children; neither were they merely filling in time. It seemed that what they were doing was deeply satisfying to them.

* * * * *

By now it must be clear to the reader that, at the Centre, the children rarely felt themselves to be the focus of the adults' attention. A child might make an appointment with his parents to come and verify his assertion that he could swim, but this would perhaps be combined with a family swim in which all were enjoying themselves together, or else, having congratulated the child on his achievement of 'the length' the parents would return to their own chosen occupations. They would show that they shared his joy and pride in his achievement but would be very unlikely to suggest to him that his next objective should be ten lengths in succession. Since the children were not organised into groups and did not want competitions or displays, there was no encouragement to the adults as such to focus their attention on the children as such, with all the possibly undesirable effects of such behaviour.

At the Centre, there was nothing to prevent the children from giving their whole attention to their present purposes and intentions and to the facts of the situation in which they were active. They were quite free of the self-consciousness that is caused by wondering if one is living up to the expectations of a parent or teacher, or indeed of a peer group with which one is involuntarily closely associated. And they were not distracted by anxiety lest they fail to achieve some external standard. Nor, strangely perhaps, considering all the glass walls, did they tend to have one eye on the spectators: they were not subject to dangers that are the result of 'showing off'. Their lack of self-consciousness enabled them to be uninterruptedly aware of what was happening around them and, in particular, of any opportunity for experience that would, at that moment, take the development of one of their faculties just a fraction further. The competitive atmosphere of school, and the self-absorption it encourages, seemed not to cling to them for one moment after they had set foot in the building.

It seems that some individuals are cursed with an excessive desire to shine in their own and other people's eyes, and with a correspondingly intense fear of failing to do so. In such a case, a person may tend to be so preoccupied with himself and with his image that he is prevented from being wholly aware of and spontaneously responsive to his surroundings. I have occasionally observed this unfortunate tendency to self-consciousness in a small child. But it can be minimised or exacerbated by his human and material environment. When small children are herded together where they are the focus of attention of adults, as they so frequently are in nurseries and playgroups, they are encouraged to be self-conscious in the worst sense of the word. The child is encouraged to look at himself through the eyes of the 'teacher' and to wonder if she approves of what he is doing. He is rarely free to watch and ponder on the life going on around him, and then, suddenly, to act; he is not free to be aware of the present state of his knowledge and knowhow and of the opportunities for learning and experience that are present and that precisely meet his needs.

It is my belief that the healthy self-esteem soon developed by the Centre children as a result of the high degree of facultisation they had achieved made them forgetful of self and therefore more aware of what was going on all around them. Certainly it was obvious that their attention was not occupied with the effect they were having and the impression they were making on people, but was directed to what they were doing and how it could best be achieved in the context of the whole situation. The fact that the adults did not make the children the centre of attention, the absence of teachers, classes, teams and competitions and overtly ambitious parents all contributed to the children's freedom from egoism.

Knowing that they were responsible for themselves and being aware of their own capacity at any time and of what was happening around them made for safety. Before the war, over a period of more than three years of free and unsupervised play in the gymnasium, there was only one serious accident, a broken arm. This was, we were told at the time, a far better record than is usual in gymnastics *classes*, where the children are under the direction and supervision of a teacher.

In *The Self-Respecting Child* I described an experience that illustrates this point:

> One day a health visitor visited our group. In our playroom a metal vice is attached to the end of the large carpenter's bench and projects beyond it, the metal handle hanging down below it at about head-height for the children. This end of the bench is close to the door so that the children must pass within two or three feet of the vice when going through the doorway. The health visitor thought that this was dangerous. I found myself surprised by her judgment because to my knowledge no child had banged himself against it in twelve years. Later, it occurred to me that in different circumstances she would have been right. If, after having been playing under the direction of a teacher for an hour or more, the children had been conducted as a party to the bathroom and had gone through the door in carefully organized single file, it would have been quite likely that one or other of them would have hurt his head against the handle of the vice. Being under orders, so to speak, they would have abdicated the responsibility for themselves and for others in favour of the teacher. They might feel that there was little point in paying careful attention to their surroundings when they had so little choice as to when, where and how they moved. They would know that the teacher did not want them to be diverted by any attractive alternative from the occupation that she had chosen for them at that moment, which was to 'go upstairs to the toilet', and they might feel that it would be less frustrating to put on blinkers, as it were, and let the teacher take the reins.

An all-age community

At the Centre, it seemed that there was an absence of the 'generation gap'. Perhaps there was no bridgeless gulf between a child and his parents, because people from other families filled it. In the child's eyes, his parents took their place in a continuum of ages in which he also saw himself. At the Centre, the emotions of the children and adolescents could be stirred by the innocent lovableness of the toddler and the courage and humour of the old, and their interest could be aroused by the unique individuality – and quirks and eccentricities – of all. Since children are motivated to learn by imitation, they are usually naturally observant, and, when they have the chance to watch undisturbed, can learn a great deal about people and situations. The Centre children could select for themselves, from among the older children, adolescents and adults young and old, those with whom they wished to become better acquainted. It was particularly easy for them to get to know their parents' friends and acquaintances, and the children of all ages, and they did not have to wait to be introduced to get a word of helpful advice from some older enthusiast for one of the activities available in the Centre. It was noticed that a particularly accomplished young man or woman might attract at times a little group of admirers.

Mutual appreciation and understanding between the adults and the children was made easier by the fact that the adults, when they were in the Centre, were also engaged in amusing themselves and in growing. Like the children, they were creating themselves; they were developing their talents and skills; they were playing.

As we have seen, the children acquired many different skills through watching others and then trying on their own. Watching what they chose to watch was always, at the Centre, an extremely important activity. They became so responsibly and happily attentive that the adults found no difficulty in allowing some of the older ones into, for instance, the 'theatre' to watch (at close quarters) the badminton or the very skilled ballroom dancing at the weekly 'Tuppenny Hop' or to watch rehearsals of the drama group. Mrs Purser has told how she remembers some older children becoming willing assistants behind the scenes to the group of adults currently working on a play or 'concert party'. The small billiards table used by the children was only a few feet away from the full-sized tables, but this did not deter the children from using it and (of course) watching the adults' game; nor did the adults object to the proximity of the children. After the first few chaotic months, the children behaved in a civilised manner and were expected by their elders to do so. When, very occasionally, one or two did not, the adults were shocked, so much so that after 40 years Bunny Arnold remembered that some children carved their initials on a table top.*

---

* See Chapter 7

At the Centre, it was not possible, as it was of old in villages and even in towns, for children to watch the cobbler, blacksmith or other craftsman at work, to stand transfixed with admiration at his skill, to identify with him and so become infected with his industry, single-mindedness and pride in a job well done; but they could be impressed by similar qualities in the amateur musician, dancer, athlete, dressmaker or conversationalist. They could also observe their parents and others enjoying the hard work of preparing for the frequent social events, parties, dances and entertainments. They had the example of adults working for a common end and could often join in if they wished.

By being in this way active and attentive on the fringe of the adults' activity, they had the opportunity to learn, without realising it, the art of social intercourse and successful co-operation.

The Centre children had another very great educational advantage: they had the chance to develop independence of mind, for common sense suggests that if a child who reaches the stage when he feels the need to think and feel independently of his parents has friends of all ages, he will be less likely to follow blindly what he imagines is the prevailing teenage philosophy and more likely to absorb bits – selected by himself – of the wisdom of older individuals, and thus become more capable of independent judgement.

There is increasing dissatisfaction with the job schools are doing. In my view, one of the reasons for this is that too much is expected of them. A great deal of a child's necessary education cannot be obtained in school, either in the classroom or on the playing fields, for a child needs to serve an apprenticeship in living.

He needs, for example, to have the experience of being a useful member of a group with which he is participating voluntarily in shared activity, the value and purpose of which he appreciates. Probably the ideal situation is when children can help their parents in a small way with making the family living, as on a small farm or market garden, a small business or workshop, when the children are not exploited but willingly give their help. For, in such cases, they can feel that they are contributing to the well-being of the family as well as gaining desired skills and powers.

In every family this can happen to a certain extent. Unfortunately, the age at which children are most keen to imitate Mum and Dad and help with the chores is often very early, when they are so little that – particularly in this age of mechanisation – great ingenuity must be exercised in order to make it possible for them to help at all effectively. My grandson of 16 months wants to try to do everything he sees his parents doing. John Holt writes*:

> In recent months I have come to know, in one case through letters, in
> another through a personal meeting, two mothers of children who, since

* In his introduction to the US edition of *The Self-Respecting Child*

before they were two, have been cooking, on a real stove, real food that they and their parents then ate. To do this, these tiny children had to move chairs to the sink or stove, and then climb on them to put water in a pot or do the cooking itself. For all my deep respect for the seriousness and ability of children, I would not have thought this possible for children under five. Such examples, of which there are probably many others, show clearly not only that children are able to be far more competent and careful than we think but also that they need far more opportunities than we give them not just for adventurous play but for serious work. From a very early age they want and need, not just to explore, but to help, to fit in, to take part, to be and feel useful and needed.

J D Hadfield writes* that in his experience, 'at three or four, children are little men and women – or want to be. Perhaps that is the time when they should be allowed to help with the chores and get the feeling of sharing usefully in work for the common well-being.' 'Four to seven', he says, 'is above all the age of independence and individuality', and seven to eleven 'the primitive man age'. As a parent and observer of children, I have found there is some truth in this. Perhaps if these general traits in children are respected and scope allowed for their fulfilment, they will be less inclined to lose their desire to practise being useful members of society and their consciousness of being capable of it.

An all-age community such as came about at the Centre can give children the opportunity to exercise their instinct to model themselves on their elders whenever it may arise, and can offer plenty of choice of models. As we have seen, it gave the four to seven year olds independence up to a point. Both in cities and in our countryside, organised as it is for specialised agriculture and motor transport, children have little chance to explore on their own and exercise responsibility for themselves, camp or make camp fires, and form gangs which devise and employ a secret language, passwords and signs. (If the latter activities were enjoyed in childhood, perhaps grown men would find them less attractive.)

After appraising the policy being adopted at the time, of attempting to deal with actual or potential anti-social adolescents by segregating them and providing them with trained leaders, Pearse and Crocker write:

It is forgotten that the natural leaders of the young are to be found in society, where every skilled man, every amateur athlete, every happily married couple, become automatically and – most important – unconsciously their leaders.[†]

The 'community schools' of Leicestershire and other places have been attempting to enable children to observe people of all ages acquiring knowledge and practising skills for the love of it. For the same reason, an Adult Education Officer of my acquaintance has nursed the ambition

* In *Childhood and Adolescence*
† 1943, p. 270

to introduce adults who are wishing to study for 'O' levels into the classes of the 14 to 16 year olds in the comprehensive school in his area. Perhaps if this sort of thing could be achieved on a large scale, teaching in schools might become more effective and discipline less of a problem.

However, in a school situation, children can only get to know and learn from adults to a limited extent. Children may love and admire a teacher and try to model themselves on him, but they do not have the opportunity to see him being himself in relation to other adults or babies or the members of his family. They do not know him in the round, as he behaves in real life situations, at home or with his friends.

Much is, or used to be, made of the 'team spirit' that was cultivated in schools. I felt when I was at school, and still feel, that 'team spirit' is not all that it is cracked up to be. For one thing, being put into teams encourages competitiveness rather than a love of doing something to the best of one's ability because one feels it is worth doing. Teachers organise children into teams in order to spur them on to make an effort; presumably it is considered that children do not, in general, want to try hard to improve their knowledge or skill and therefore need an extra incentive. Probably teachers feel that they cannot be continually urging a child to 'beat' his companions, whereas they can encourage him to help his team to 'beat' another team with a clear conscience. Any form of competition can be quite fun to a child whose talents lie in the required direction but, to the others, the prospect – or the memory – of letting the team down can be hell.

It was not until as an adult addressing envelopes with other members of a political party on the eve of an election that I remember experiencing – with surprise – a feeling of joy in shared effort for a shared purpose.

Jean Liedloff expresses what I am trying to say very well. When she was living with the Yequana in the Venezuelan jungle and had walked several miles over rough and mountainous country to buy some sugar cane for herself, she found that on the return journey her two Amerindian companions expected her to carry a small part of the load. This, she wrote, she would previously have found an unbearable imposition and she was on the point of refusing to carry the one heavy cane they had allotted to her as her share. Luckily, having a great admiration for the good sense and wisdom of one of the Indians, she decided to try, and lifted the cane and balanced it on her shoulder. Very soon she found that the two men's good humoured enjoyment of the journey had entirely dispelled the feelings of strain, hurry and competition and the sense of being a martyr that had always assailed her previously when carrying a load in the company of Europeans, over similar country.

> Then a new pleasure added itself to my freedom: I was aware of carrying not just a stick of cane but part of a load shared among three

companions. I had heard about 'team spirit' until it ceased to connote anything but pretence at school and summer camp. One's own position had always been at risk. One was always threatened, watched, judged. The straightforward business of doing a task in partnership with a fellow-being was lost in a tangle of competitiveness; the primordial feeling of pleasure at pooling one's forces with those of others had never had a chance to arise.*

Perhaps experience of this primordial pleasure can be a means of developing in children their ability to be truly social and responsible and nourish their desire to be useful and creative members of society.

Many of the member-families became aware that the Centre was a healthy place of education for their children. Their strong desire and successful efforts to have their own Centre school is evidence of this. Some were also aware that the children were promoting the health of their families. 'Children keep you young,' they said. Scott Williamson said, 'Children are the fastest growing-points of the family organism,' and can be the main means of its 'growth and differentiation'; they can contribute increasingly to the growth of the 'home'. It became possible for Centre families to be wholes composed of individually growing and free parts – as he said, 'free but not loose parts'.

The Centre demonstrated that when parents and children are both parts of the life of a local neighbourhood community, even the small modern 'nuclear' family is able to perform the family's two main biological functions – the nurture of new, unique individualities and the development of maturity in all the members of the family, both children and parents.

Reverence for life

The value which the Peckham Biologists attached to the family and the care they took to extend any information they had to give to both partners, thus involving them both in any decision concerning the family, played a large part in making the Centre into a family club in fact as well as in name. Another very important factor was the integration of the children into the society of the adults. Each child and adolescent as well as each adult could – and did – contribute to and profit from the diversity and richness of the community life of the Centre.

This had come about because the Peckham Biologists treated each child with no less respect than they accorded their parents. Scott Williamson's call for greater humility, his adjuration to people to take a more humble attitude towards life and all its manifestations, was not mere rhetoric. He and his closest colleagues were imbued with the humble spirit of a true biologist. And they were honest and clear sighted. If, they reasoned, the necessary conditions for the emergence of health in adults were what they suspected them to be, children must need them

* 1975

too; if adults needed the opportunity to be the directors of their own lives, so did children – in all the areas in which a child is capable of good judgement. This and their faith in the biological wisdom of a healthy child were, I believe, crucial factors among those that made it possible for the Centre to become a community created and enjoyed by all the family, and a place where health could flower.

Chapter 11

A New Concept of Health

Scott Williamson and Innes Pearse wrote of the Pioneer Health Centre:

> The Centre is the first experimental station in human biology. It asks the question – what circumstances will sustain human beings in their capacity for full function (i.e. in health); and what orientation will such fully functioning entities give to human living (i.e. to society)?

One way of trying to find the answers to these questions is to make considered and reasoned conjectures as to the basic physical and social environmental circumstances in which people may cultivate health, attempt to create these circumstances and then find out if they do, in fact, have that effect. One may find that some of them are right and some are wrong, and have to change or modify the circumstances accordingly. Obviously it is impossible to start out on such an experimental course without having some sort of an idea of what health is; one must have already formed a preliminary concept of the nature of health, in order to be able to make sensible guesses of the nature of the circumstances in which a person may cultivate it in himself and in his society, and to be able to judge the value of these guesses.

Scott Williamson had been reflecting on the subject of positive health all his working life, and by the time he came to plan the main experiment in the early 1930s, he had arrived at a tentative theory of the nature of health and of the basic needs of human beings if they are to be healthy. During the experiment, he confirmed his basic theory to his own satisfaction, but he also modified and developed it, as observation deepened his understanding. This chapter contains the result of my personal mental digestion of Scott Williamson's theory – or hypothesis, as he preferred to call it.

His hypothesis seems revolutionary, yet it is firmly based on certain common sense facts. The first of these is that a person is a living being, an organism – however many characteristics he may possess that are not shared by other species. The second is that an organism possesses certain attributes that distinguish it from a mere aggregation of bits of inorganic matter like a rock or a drop of water. Three of these attributes are uniqueness, wholeness and the power of creative growth.

If asked point blank, zoologists and other students of the 'life sciences' would, I believe, accept these assumptions as valid, although, in their work and their theories, they may ignore them.

1. **Uniqueness*** – Well-known pieces of evidence of this in humans are fingerprints, handwriting and the tendency of the body to reject bits of another person's body that a surgeon has tried to graft on to it. Surgeons have discovered how to overcome this resistance to foreign bodies by the use of drugs to some extent, but, if one needs a skin graft for example, it is better to provide the piece of skin oneself. Every part of the body partakes of this uniqueness.

It is not only the anatomy and the tissues and the cells (old and new) of the body that are peculiar to a particular person. His movements and gestures, his posture and the way he walks are also specific to him. One can recognise a person by the sound of his step or his voice, or by the turn of phrase or the vocabulary he uses: his behaviour is unique as well as his body. Furthermore, a person can be recognised by his artifacts and creations. The signature, as it were, of a painter, potter, musician or writer is apparent in their works. Lovers of the arts can correctly name the composer of a piece of music they have never heard before or the creator of a piece of sculpture, a painting or drawing that they see for the first time.

As we have seen, Piaget holds that a baby begins at birth to choose what it will attend to out of the kaleidoscope of sensory stimulation in which it is immersed. Then, from the information it receives from the events, materials, objects and forces that it chooses to attend to, it builds up its own unique body of knowledge. From the beginning, it proceeds to create its own special picture of the world.

So every baby's view of the world is different from that of any other, and, as anyone can observe, every baby not only looks quite different from any other baby but responds to the world in a manner that is special to him.

2. **Wholeness** – One of the meanings of the word 'organism' given in the Penguin English Dictionary is 'organised structure of parts working together for the existence of the whole'. This is, in my opinion, a more complete meaning of the word than those given in other dictionaries. A plant or an animal is composed of definable units each of which has its particular part to play in the maintenance and functioning of the whole plant or animal. When healthy, each of these parts – organs, tissues, cells – behaves in awareness of the needs of the whole – or so it seems; and the whole organism, if it obeys its instincts, acts in apparent awareness of the needs of its parts. The whole tends to behave in a way that ensures the well-being and efficiency of the parts and the parts do what promotes the well-being and efficiency of the whole. Smuts, discussing the relationship between cells and organisms, writes:

> Look for instance, at the way in which organisms behave when some cells or organs, necessary for their maintenance, are removed or injured.

* For an eye opener on this, read Williams, 1967

It is well known that many plants and animals have the power of restitution in case of damage or mutilation. The newt forms a new leg in the place of the severed limb. The plant supplies the place of the severed branch with another. The regeneration may be effected from different organs and by different organs. Thus if the crystalline lens is removed from the eye of a Triton, the iris will regenerate a new lens, although the lens and the iris in this case have been evolved from quite different parts. Numerous similar curious facts of restoration could be mentioned. The broken whole in organic nature restores itself or is restored by the undamaged parts. The cells of the remaining parts set themselves the novel task of restoring the missing parts. The power to do this varies with various plants or animals, and varies also with the different parts in the same plant or animal. Generally one may say that the more highly differentiated and specialised an organism or a cell is, the smaller is its plasticity, or the power of the remaining cells to restore the whole in case of injury or mutilation. But the fact that the power exists in numerous cases is a proof that not only can the cells through reproduction build up the original organism according to its specific type, but also that when this type is damaged the remaining cells or some of them can restore it, and recomplete the whole. The normal power of the cells to build up an organism in reproduction according to type is one thing, and it is marvellous enough even though one looks upon it as merely a case of inherited routine. But the abnormal power to do this in the very unusual case, so far removed from all idea of routine, where the type is broken down is something different, and shows how effective is the power of the organism as a whole, and how strong is the tendency towards the whole in the individual cells. The damage creates a need, and the need stimulates the remaining parts to perform the functions of the damaged parts or to restore them in whole or in part. The very nature of the cells is to function as parts of a whole, and when the whole is broken down an unusual extra task automatically arises for them to restore the breach, and their dormant powers are aroused to action. And this happens, so far as we can see, simply as a matter of interior economy and domestic regulation in the organism itself and without previous education for the new role. The interaction between the organism and its cells is indeed most subtle and intimate, both seem to be active factors in the maintenance of the whole and in the restoration of any parts that may be missing and necessary for the whole. So intimate is their interaction that it is almost impossible to say where the influence of the one ends and the other begins...

The organism is indeed a little living world in which law and order reign, and in which every part collaborates with every other part, and subserves the common purposes of the whole, as a rule with the most perfect regularity.

But the individual cell does not lose its own identity:

The organism embraces innumerable smaller organic units whose identity is not swallowed up in it, is expressed and not suppressed by it. The large organism does not only mean the union and co-operative harmony of its smaller units, but also as a rule the more perfect individuation and specialised development of these units in the harmony of the whole. The plant or animal body is a social community, but a community which allows a substantial development to its individual members. And its nature and structure are such that it can only perfect itself through the differentiation and development of the members which compose it.*

He says that an organic whole is more than merely the sum of its parts, yet it contains nothing in addition to them; it is not something super-imposed on them. 'It *is* the parts in their unity: it is a synthesis of the parts.' This synthesis has a special character, a unique individuality which pervades each part and every activity of part and whole.

3. **The power of creative growth** – A living being has the power to grow, not by the addition of similar material as happens to a snowball when it is rolled over the snow, but by the *digestion* of elements of its environment. If suitably nourishing material finds its way into a body's digestive system and other conditions are favourable, the parts of the body specialised for the purpose break down the food into elements that can be transported around the body to where they are needed. Then the body and its parts select items of this material and use them to build and restore themselves and, in the process, they *transform* them into material that is quite different from the original food material. The process is known as metabolism. The material that, as a result of this process, has become a part of the body is not only different in character from what it was before, it also bears that body's own unique stamp: each new skin, bone or hair cell is characteristic of that particular body. Since each body is different from any other body past or present, what is built is new – original. So physical growth and renewal are creative processes. How-ever, a body does not create from nothing; it transforms *existing material* into something new: it recombines and reorganises substances. It synthesises; and the resulting material is both new, and specific to that body. Smuts referred to this process as creative synthesis.

Scott Williamson also used the word synthesis to describe the means by which healthy living beings grow, but he qualified it by the adjective 'subjective'. He did this in order to prevent confusion with the more usual meaning of the word when it is used with reference to the actions of humans, the intentional combination of substances in the production of new substances, which is an objective synthesis.

Since a person is a whole, an indivisible unit of life, it is reasonable to assume that his physical and mental powers and his knowledge grow by a process similar to metabolism. It is reasonable to assume that they grow in the same way as the body, by the selection, digestion, and synthesis of elements of the environment. As we have seen, Jean Piaget's lengthy and intensive research has provided plenty of evidence

* 1926

that supports this assumption. To Smuts it was a self-evident fact. 'Creative synthesis is characteristic of all organic actions and functions.' Man's potentiality for creative synthesis is far greater than that of other organisms but it arises in the same manner as 'the novelty and initiative which we see in organic Nature'.*

We speak of 'food for thought' and of a person having 'digested' a book, an experience, or a piece of information in the sense of having thoroughly assimilated it and integrated it into his own mental furniture and of having, if necessary, reorganised or adjusted his mental furniture to fit it. These commonly used expressions are surely evidence that people have long taken it for granted that the process of growth is similar in body and in mind.

> Inanimate nature obeys the Second Law of Thermodynamics (it decreases in its degree of organisation, becoming more and more run-down). Life by contrast is inherently synthetic. It manufactures new organic compounds of bewildering variety. The key of the process is organisation... The organising capacity of life is not confined to chemical synthesis. Organisms adapt, reproduce, invent and grow in a manner unknown to inanimate nature... The living person continually synthesises foodstuffs, oxygen, bacterial action, past experiences, present needs and images of the future. By so doing he not only survives as an independent being but develops and grows in such a way as to become ever more characteristic of what he is.†

Summing up what has so far been said in this chapter, the three attributes, wholeness, unique individuality and the power to grow by means of the subjective synthesis of elements of the environment are characteristic of a fully functioning organism – an organism that is functioning healthily. Since a person is an organism, he will, if he is healthy, share these attributes. They are as characteristic of health in humans as in all other forms of life.

It was manifestations of these three characteristics of health that Scott Williamson hoped to see in the subjects of his enquiry. As will now be evident to the reader, he was interested in what people do, *not* in what he or anyone else – or they themselves – thought they ought to do. With his biological outlook, he was aware always of the relationship of a person with his material and social environment. So, he aimed to create the environmental conditions that would make it possible for people to be fully functioning, and then see what happened.

In conditions that are inappropriate for healthy growth, humans may behave like a hibernating animal. A better anology than this and the one used by the Peckham Biologists, is a body cell that builds a defensive wall around itself, forming a cyst; the cell continues to exist but ceases to function. In conditions that are unsuitable for health, people may be surviving in an encysted state – not fully living.

* 1926
† Allport, 1937

Scott Williamson's genius was practical as well as theoretical. Others have postulated that healthily functioning living beings manifest properties such as these, but Williamson actually created a situation in which the kind of conditions people need to experience if they are to live fully, can emerge.

He saw that one of the most necessary of these is continuity of acquaintanceship with others: man is a social species; a person cannot develop his full humanity and wisdom in isolation. If he is to be healthy, his environment, for at least a part of his life, must contain other people. Nor can people form the kind of human relationships they need if they are drifting through an amorphous and shifting crowd. A person needs to be a distinct and effective member of a more or less stable group, and to have such a group as a base camp from which to make expeditions into the unknown. For children this is particularly necessary; they need the opportunity to attach themselves to a few special people and to make themselves thoroughly familiar with their own special territory – their home. This fact was not generally recognised in the thirties. Only quite recently has it been discovered that children who have no family of their own are better off in someone else's than in an institution with a crowd of others and changing care givers, and that babies reared in hospital conditions do not usually thrive. The Centre with its neighbourhood and family membership provided opportunity for the 'continuity of association with others' that, the Peckham Biologists realised, people need. The family membership also ensured a diversity in the environment of the members that was due to the presence of individuals of all stages of maturity.

Mutual synthesis of part and whole

The faculty to be oneself, to act as an integrated, unique and growing whole was, to Scott Williamson, essential to health. Through being himself and, at the same time, being aware of as much as is possible of the whole of his surroundings, including events and people, and responding spontaneously to this whole, he makes the contribution only he can make to the social whole of which he is a part; and the whole is enriched. This is in addition to the quantity of the benefits that his talents, skills and inventiveness may bring to a group or community. It lies in the personal quality of his behaviour, in the 'specificity of his action-pattern'.

Williamson saw that it is not only that one individual influences another within a social whole; it is that the environment that the whole provides receives *from* each individual the unique effects of his growth and, as a result, offers *to* each individual a greater choice of 'nourishment', and thus a greater opportunity to satisfy his unique growth-needs. The part and the whole, the person and the group, are in a mutually nourishing and fertilising relationship. He called it a 'relationship of mutual synthesis'. He wrote that the nearest he could get to a definition of health is a *'progressive mutual synthesis participated in by both organism and environment'*.

In *The Peckham Experiment*, Pearse and Crocker write:

> Take, for example, a pollen grain dropped on a membrane of an animal's body. It is drawn into the tissues of that body, where it is engulfed and digested by a wandering leucocyte, so adding its quota to the body metabolism. This is not different from a process that can be seen in the environment when a leaf or a petal falls on the ground, whence the earthworm drags it down into the earth, there to digest and remove it, and in so doing provides essential nutrient for the society of the soil population. Both the body of the living entity and the 'body' of the environment are recipients of the respective digest, each entity changing the material in a manner specific to its kind before its incorporation into new life. As there is a metabolism of any living entity, so there is a 'metabolism' of the body of the environment: each takes and each gives...
>
> Thus, the environment is the source of diversity as well as the recipient of the diversification of that which is taken from it by the organism. Each different factor or change in the environment that impinges on the organism, each new food particle digested, each new co-ordination learned as a result of experience made possible by any new environmental disposition, results in the development of further specificity in the organism and leads to a still more versatile power of apprehension of further environmental contributions. Also, and consequently, it leads to still further novelty in the products subsequently received into the environment. So that in the presence of adequate nutriment, function implies an ever increasing diversification, in the organism and in the environment alike...*

The word 'function' was given a special meaning by Scott Williamson which made it a useful piece of shorthand. He used it to mean the kind of activity – mental, physical or social – which is healthy because it promotes the development of a person's fullest capacities and, as a result, enriches his life and the social and physical environment he shares with others.

> Here then is a picture not of hostility between the organism and its environment but of mutuality at work in the living world. Yet hitherto the development and indeed the very existence of the organism has been pictured by the scientist as a 'struggle for survival'; while Man in his acknowledged supremacy is alleged to have conquered Nature, rather than to have wooed her in the sensitivity of a mutual – or loving – relationship.†

It is now more frequently recognised that, in nature undisturbed by man, a species and its ecosystem (or immediate bit of the biosphere) are

* 1965, pp. 27–8
† 1943, p. 24

mutually dependent and, usually, mutually beneficial or they would not continue to co-exist. Each species has found what ecologists call a 'niche' in the ecosystem, each (with a few exceptions – nature may be orderly but it is not neat and tidy) contributes to the welfare of the ecosystem as a whole during its life or by its death.

> The mutual action of organism and environment, associated as we rise in the biological scale with an increasing degree of autonomy in the organism, recalls forcibly to mind the circumstances of a single cell, such, for instance, as the liver cell, set in the body of which it is an infinitesimal part. The cell acts as liver cell carrying on the specific function of 'liverness', yet always, in health, 'aware' of and subject to the wider needs of the body of which it is a part and from which it derives sustenance. It is this relationship to the body which alone gives significance to its individuality as liver cell as well as to its unique function of liverness... Can it be that Man himself is but a cell in the body of Cosmos; and that Cosmos is organismal as he is?*

Observation of the operation of mutual synthesis of part and whole throughout nature and within each organism led Scott Williamson to envisage 'cosmos' as living – as 'one organic whole'; 'the total environment and the organisms it contains constitute one organic unity.' This idea does not seem so extraordinary today as it may have done in his time. Theodore Roszak has written:

> Within less than a generation, thoughtful people around the world begin to see that nature must have its natural rights; the rights of the planet to its self-sustaining integrity, its native dignity.†

In 1979, J E Lovelock FRS published a book in which he put forward what has come to be called the 'Gaia hypothesis'. He writes:

> The physical and chemical condition of the surface of the Earth, of the atmosphere, and of the oceans has been – and is – actively made fit and comfortable by the presence of life itself... The entire range of living matter on Earth, from whales to viruses and from oaks to algae, could be regarded as constituting a single living entity, capable of manipulating the Earth's atmosphere to suit its overall needs and endowed with faculties and powers far beyond those of its constituent parts.

Not only are the proportions of the gases composing the Earth's atmosphere quite different from those contained in the atmospheres of other planets but they have been maintained in a certain – and very subtle – balance for millions of years.

> The chemical composition of the atmosphere bears no relation to the expectations of steady-state chemical equilibrium. The presence of methane, nitrous oxide, and even nitrogen in our present oxidizing atmosphere represents violation of the rules of chemistry to be measured in tens of orders of magnitude. Disequilibria on this scale suggest that the

* 1943
† 1977

atmosphere is not merely a biological product, but more probably a biological construction: not living, but like a cat's fur, a bird's feathers, or the paper of a wasp's nest, an extension of a living system designed to maintain a chosen environment. Thus the atmospheric concentration of gases such as oxygen and ammonia is found to be kept at an optimum value from which even small departures could have disastrous consequences for life...

We have since defined Gaia as a complex entity involving the Earth's biosphere, atmosphere, oceans, and soil; the totality constituting a feedback or cybernetic system which seeks an optimal physical and chemical environment for life on this planet. The maintenance of relatively constant conditions by active control may be conveniently described by the term 'homoeostasis'.*

Lovelock warns that Gaia can compensate for or repair the damage done to her constitution by man's irresponsible behaviour only up to a point. He cites tropical forests, the wetlands and the shallow seas close to the continental shores as the places in which the most serious and irrevocable damage could be done. He is not in favour of trying to put the clock back: he holds that science and technology can and must be used to help combat the harm that has been done to the biosphere by the indiscriminate and careless use of technology.

It was part of Scott Williamson's hypothesis that within the ultimate all-encompassing organic whole there are many lesser wholes – wholes within wholes – of which a living being may be part and with which he may be in a relationship of mutual synthesis. One of the wholes instanced by the Peckham Biologists is that formed by mother and foetus – 'the pregnancy'.

Here mother and foetus are linked into a unity by a special organ – the placenta – newly formed for that purpose, and built into a wall of the womb by their joint operations, both of them contributing to its substance and to its construction. It is through the selective membranes of this placenta that the many and varied contents of the maternal blood and lymph reach the foetus, there to be built up into its organised substance under the unified control of 'the pregnancy'. It is through the membranes of the placenta equally, that pass the substances from the foetus which stir further developmental changes in the maternal body and at the same time lead to preparation of the food necessary to the child when born.†

Another is the family, which they define as a woman and a man in a continuing and growing relationship – with or without children. They held that the family (woman plus man) is the complete human organism, and only through the birth and growth of this organism can individuals fully realise their potential maturity.

When two diverse individuals function as an organism, *all that they encounter* acquires a new significance. It is not merely the addition of the

---

* Lovelock, 1979
† 1943, p. 140

experience of one to that of the other, making the combined view a larger whole seen, but that with a new polarity a new *quality* is given to their apprehension. And this quality of perception is given not only to what is experienced at the moment, but that experience itself influences what they in their new functional orientation will in the future experience – hence altering their every action.*

Examples of communities in which the mutual synthesis of person and group occurred, such as the hunting band of the Pygmies or the village or street communities of the past, are described in the present book, also examples of temporary wholes in which it can occur such as groups of playing children.

A central implication of Scott Williamson's theory of the nature of health is that crippled or disabled children or adults can be healthy; they can have a healthy appetite for experience and can develop fully their potential capability. As a result, they can be aware and responsible to the limit of their capacity and, through acting effectively, can enjoy a feeling of self-confidence and self-esteem. No doubt others besides myself will recall examples of this. I have described one in *The Self-Respecting Child* (chapter 10).

Useful instincts

Scott Williamson and Pearse wrote, (1949):

By the study of health is implied study of the unfolding of the fullest human capacities.

As we have seen, they held that a healthy child is biologically motivated from birth to do what he needs to do in order to develop his essential human capacities. He has an instinct to develop his human faculties through the digestion and synthesis of experience. If his physical and social environment consistently provides him with the opportunity for action that promotes human growth and development, the instinct will be likely to persist, although, since everyone is unique, it may be stronger in some than in others.

I am told that, if I want to be taken seriously by present-day students of the Life Sciences (especially psychologists and sociologists) I must avoid, when discussing human beings, the use of the word 'instinct'. If I do not, those who adhere to the 'blank sheet' theory or those who, like the Existentialists, cherish a belief in the total freedom of a person to be exactly what he chooses to be, will immediately write me off as hopelessly out of date, if not reactionary.

Mary Midgley† says that a part of the trouble is an either/or attitude: people still range themselves on one or other side of the old 'Nature versus Nurture' controversy. This hoary battle has become exacerbated by actual or imputed political alignments and so it has become more

* 1943, p. 19
† 1979

difficult to bury the hatchet and get down to some realistic and constructive thinking. Common sense surely indicates that what a person *is* at any moment is determined *both* by his past environment and by his genes and, above all, by what he himself has felt, pondered on and done throughout his life – by what he has chosen to attend to, respond to and in what manner he has responded. But common sense does not seem to be much used in places of higher education. As if they were playing the children's game of Oranges and Lemons, people think they are called on to opt for one side or the other and, as Midgley says, 'either be loyal innatists or faithful environmentalists'. She helps to clear away the cloud of dust kicked up by this quite unnecessary and futile tug-of-war by distinguishing between 'closed' and 'open' instincts.*

When instinct is used in the latter sense, human beings may be said to have an instinct to care for children, an instinct to learn the art of forming rewarding and stable relationships with others, or an instinct to behave in ways that will exercise and develop their human capabilities to the full. Instinctive tendencies such as these are a part of human nature. The instincts to propagate, to care for their young, and to behave in a way that is necessary in order to become competent must have been essential for the survival of any living species during all the time there was life on the Earth. As most anthropologists today agree, it is to be expected that behaviour tending to lead to the formation of rewarding and stable relationships with others would have become instinctive in humans because Homo Sapiens depended for its biological success on the ability to co-operate and to live in stable groups. Without this, our ancestors would not have been able to care effectively for their exceptionally slowly-maturing young, nor to prey on game of all kinds, including animals much larger, swifter or better armoured than themselves, and on which they depended not only for food but also for material for shelter, clothing, weapons and tools. If early men and women had not possessed these abilities, they would not have successfully colonised so much of the surface of the world.

If biologists are right in stating that the period of civilisation has been too short to affect the basic genetic structure of the human species, we must have within us – if buried more or less deeply – the same helpful 'open instincts' that were possessed by our human ancestors for thousands of generations.

* * * * *

The faculty for choice

The Peckham Biologists used the word 'instinct' rarely – probably aware of its ambiguity – and always in the singular. They preferred 'involuntary or autonomic wisdom'. As an example of this kind of wisdom, they

---

* See Chapter 7 above

cite the behaviour of the embryo – the way it grows and develops according to the pattern or 'promise' contained in its genes. At birth, the baby does not lose the instinctive or biological wisdom, that guided him in the womb. As long as his environment continues to be suitable for healthy growth, he will tend to do what he needs to do in order to continue to grow healthily and develop fully; he behaves as he needs to behave if his potential faculties are to develop fully. He exercises what the Peckham Biologists called 'the faculty for choice'. This faculty, they postulated, is an essential attribute of health – 'In health we choose what meets our needs.'

If we are to get their meaning, we must rid our minds of the idea that the word 'choice' inevitably implies the making of conscious decisions. When using the word in the Peckham sense, it is correct to say that the body chooses the particular elements of the food in its stomach that it needs at any moment for energy, maintenance and growth. To say merely that it 'takes' these elements is inadequate for it takes only certain elements; it discriminates; it selects.

Jean Liedloff's experience of the Yequana people* may help to clarify the Peckham Biologists' meaning of the phrase 'faculty for choice'. At the least, it may prevent anyone from getting the false impression that it is an esoteric power only attainable by saints and mystics.

Piaget has shown that a baby whose environment is suitable chooses spontaneously – instinctively – biologically, from the very beginning, the precise bits of knowledge and knowhow that are presently needed for the nourishment of his mental and sensory-motor faculties. It seemed to me that most of the children in the Centre and in my playgroup were doing this and, moreover, that they were also choosing the experiences they needed for the growth of their power of discrimination, their judgement, emotional power and love of life. In the process, their faculty to choose according to their needs – to choose rightly – was strengthening. Like all faculties, the faculty for choice requires exercise if it is to grow and develop. If the kind of conditions in which it can operate are never present, it will, like a muscle that is never used, become weak and finally wither away.

How can we discover what these conditions are, so that we may provide them for our children, and they may grow up to be wiser than we are? The first step is to accept and thoroughly digest the idea that humans are born with an instinct to choose rightly for themselves and that, therefore, our best teachers are babies and small children themselves.

We may also learn from peoples who have lived for centuries in a close relationship with nature. There are small pockets of people, mainly hidden away in the depths of forests, who appear to have successfully cultivated the faculty for choice in themselves and their children, and to

* See Chapter 9 above

have learned how to live happily and effectively in families and larger groups, and in mutual synthesis with their environment as a whole. We shall have to hurry, for the forest is being destroyed or its inhabitants seduced by the superficial advantages of industrial civilisation. Some of those who have decided that their own traditional way of life is better have retreated into more inhospitable country (for instance, in tropical South America, nearer to the summits of the forest-clad mountains where life is harder but undisturbed) and do not welcome visitors from the cities. We would do well to make the most of what has already been observed by the few travellers and anthropologists who have succeeded in obtaining the trust and confidence of such peoples.*

According to the Peckham Biologists, the faculty for choice functions fully – or can function fully – in the phenomenon of falling in love: 'in health, we choose the right mate.'

> Even in homo sapiens Nature does not leave mating to chance or wholly to man's choice, for falling in love – herald of the process – is an instinctive and involuntary, or autonomic happening. An individual may of volition attempt to stay its consequences; he cannot prevent or anticipate its advent. And, when men and women do fall in love, they are precipitated into a stream of events which in many an instance leads them into paths they had no intention of exploring. This urge to biological completion of the human organism is of immense potency, its strength and delicacy fully comparable to anything yet encountered in the dynamic field. It can move an individual from one end of the earth to the other; can uproot men and women from the binding tentacles of habit and change the tenor of their lives; can release unsuspected potentialities and endow action with immeasurable fortitude...
>
> In health or wholeness, the bias of sex in man and woman is brought naturally to balance in the unity of the family ... Sex is the means Nature uses to bring man and woman to adulthood and to the full participation in her life process, for sex is the very basis of creative or evolutionary energy.†

Diversity

It is probable that, at its beginning, life made several false starts. It is certain that many species have become extinct through failing to cope with natural catastrophes and climatic changes; but there was always sufficient diversity in the forms of life on the Earth for new species to take their place. The uniqueness of every organism has resulted in a diversity that has ensured the stability of life.

In the same way, the more individuality – and resultant diversity – there is in a human society, the more stable it is likely to be. For example, the more individual people are – the more they think for themselves and develop their own power of judgement, follow their own

---

* I have described some of their observations in Chapter 9 above. See also Thomas, 1959, Donner, 1984 and others.
† 1943, Chapter 12, Courtship and Mating

feelings and tastes and exercise their faculty for choice – the less likely it is that they will be slaves to fashion with its tendency to swing to extremes and tip the baby out with the bathwater, or that they will line up behind leaders and join warring factions. There are less likely to be violent or wholesale changes and more likely to be a gradual evolution in the same way as in the natural world where any alteration has to prove its worth or it will not prevail against the resistance to change and conservatism of nature.

It is when individuality is developed in a few people only, that it can be dangerous to society as a whole; for then there is a greater danger of changes occurring which destroy the beneficial traditions together with the bad and leave people in so much confusion that they grasp at straws which turn out to be chains, and they are worse off than they were before.

In the whole that was the Centre, there was both diversity and stability. People were able to become thoroughly well acquainted with their environment, and so were able to act with both spontaneity and realism.* The same was the case in my 'free-choice' playgroup; and, in that simple and limited situation, it was easily observable. The following is from the day-to-day notes I made and drew from to illustrate my thesis in *The Self-Respecting Child*:

> Today I suddenly realized that Caroline and her devoted admirer Sandra (aged $4^1/_4$ and 4 years respectively) had spent the whole of the morning except for three roughly ten-minute intervals – one for elevenses, one to paint a picture and one to do a jigsaw puzzle – playing on the slides, and in the course of their play had devised a new 'trick'. They had placed the two planks close together supported upon the tool-chest and had discovered how to slide, first crouching low and finally standing upright on their stockinged feet – neither shoes nor bare feet being slippery enough – in exactly the same manner as a skier descends a snow slope. In the days that followed, as one or two of the other children imitated them, the new 'trick' became one of the traditional skills of the group. It still is at the time of writing, one and a half years later, though the inventors left the group to go to school twelve months ago.

What adult would have thought of suggesting such a game or would have guessed how popular it would have remained? It was a particularly spectacular instance of the spontaneous inventiveness of the children. But in this playgroup *every* child was continuously responding in his own unique manner to his environment. He was adding to the diversity in the environment. This meant that the surroundings of each child were rich in opportunities for the growth of faculties, creativity and judgement. And, as a result, the activity was never exactly the same from day to day; what the children found good was preserved. Each child's skill was growing; ideas were being tried out,

---

* This is discussed further in the next section of this chapter.

and did not escape the notice of the other children who might or might not adopt them for their own, or be inspired by them to further creativity.

It was possible for this to happen only because the basis was stable. The children knew each other well, since I kept the fee for each session low and most of the children came every day. The material environment was also basically the same from day to day. For example, the 'slides' (two polished hardwood planks supported on a heavy carpenter's bench side by side, or, alternatively, as the children wished, on the lower 'toolchest') were in position for most of the session. Sometimes I arranged the equipment slightly differently, usually when requested to do so by a child, and very occasionally made a suggestion as to how it might be used, but the children knew that they were quite free to ignore my suggestions. (The very rare command or warning, they recognised as such because it was delivered in a different, more urgent tone of voice.) And the overall layout of the main pieces of apparatus remained the same from day to day.

As Lewis Carroll's Alice found in the garden of the King and Queen of Hearts, it is impossible to play croquet effectively in totally unfamiliar conditions. Because the children could continue from day to day to make themselves increasingly familiar with their surroundings, they quickly grew in efficacy and skills of all kinds. Each could make use of the diversity in the environment that was the result of this, for their own purposes. The changes – the diversification – were the effect of mutual synthesis of part and whole; they arose from within the whole that was the playgroup, instead of being imposed from without; and they were therefore more likely to be of a kind that was both comprehensible and inspiring to the children.

* * * *

That human health requires a diverse environment was understood by an eighteenth-century Prussian, Wilhelm von Humboldt (brother of the explorer). During his career as a government servant of his country, he wrote a book called *The Limits of State Action*. Knowing his views to be unacceptable to his compatriots, he did not publish it until later in life – in 1772. In it he wrote:

> The true end of Man, or that which is prescribed by the eternal and immutable dictates of reason, and not suggested by vague and transient desires, is the highest and most harmonious development of his powers to a complete and consistent whole. Freedom is the first and indispensable condition which the possibility of such a development presupposes; but there is besides another essential – intimately connected with freedom, it is true – a variety of situations. Even the most free and self-reliant of men is hindered in his development, when set in a monotonous situation.

But, as it is evident that *such a diversity is a constant result of freedom**
... these two conditions, of freedom and variety of situation, may be
regarded, in a certain sense, as one and the same.

John Stuart Mill took a quotation from von Humboldt as a foreword
for his famous essay *On Liberty*:

> The grand, leading principle, towards which every argument unfolded in
> these pages directly converges, is the absolute and essential importance
> of human development in its richest diversity.

Spontaneity, responsibility and autonomy

In *On Liberty*, Mill writes:

> Human nature is not a machine to be built after a model, and set to do
> the work prescribed for it, but a tree, which requires to grow and develop
> on all sides, according to the tendency of the inward forces which make
> it a living thing...
>
> It is not by wearing down into uniformity all that is individual in
> themselves, but by cultivating it and calling it forth, within the limits
> imposed by the rights and interests of others, that human beings become
> a noble and beautiful object of contemplation; and as the works partake
> the character of those who do them, by the same process human life also
> becomes rich, diversified and animating, furnishing more abundant ali-
> ment to high thoughts and elevating feelings, and strengthening the tie
> which binds every individual to the race, by making the race infinitely
> better worth belonging to. In proportion to the development of his indivi-
> duality, each person becomes more valuable to himself, and is, therefore,
> capable of being more valuable to others. There is a greater fullness of
> life about his own existence, and when there is more life in the units,
> there is more in the mass which is composed of them.

He makes a complaint that is relevant still:

> But the evil is that individual spontaneity is hardly recognised by the
> common modes of thinking as having any intrinsic worth... spontaneity
> forms no part of the ideal of the majority of moral and social reformers,
> but is rather looked on with jealousy as a troublesome and perhaps
> rebellious obstruction to the general acceptance of what these reformers,
> in their own judgment, think would be best for mankind.

Mill was aware that spontaneous action on the part of the individual
was a necessary condition both for the full development of individuality
and for diversity in the environment. By the word spontaneity, he obviously does not mean the following of any and every impulse or a
reaction to a part of the environmental circumstances only, as when one
obeys the impulse to avoid a puddle only to step into the path of an
approaching vehicle. Scott Williamson applied the term to the behaviour
of a person who is acting as an integrated whole in response to his

* My italics

understanding of the reality of the situation as a whole, in contrast to action that is a mechanical response to a particular environmental or internal stimulus or is the result of habit or prejudice.

But Scott Williamson knew that spontaneity is not enough. Another quality of activity is necessary – 'autonomy'. He gives this word a particular meaning. He uses it to mean more than the usual 'self-government'; he uses it to include the kind of behaviour displayed by healthy cells in their relationship to a healthy body. A cell acts individually – on its own initiative as it were – but also according to the unique needs of the body of which it is a part and on which it depends for sustenance.

> The pathologist is only too familiar with the situation that arises where this delicately poised relationship of the cell's autonomy within the sphere of a greater organisation – the body – is absent. When the cell multiplies without reference to the impulses of the greater organisation of the body of its inhabitation, the result is cancer, the definition of which might be stated as 'multiplication without function' – loss of individuality. Such procedure ushers in antagonism, disrupting the mutual association between the cell and its environment – and ends in the ultimate destruction of the cell, or of the body in which it grows.*

If a cell begins to act merely mechanically instead of in a sensitive relation to the body as a whole, the body may recognise it as harmful and get rid of it. (There is a current theory that it is only when the body is not healthy enough to be capable of this that cancerous cells can flourish, spread and take over.)

In health, the cell or organ acts as an 'autonomous' part of the body as a whole. It is free to be its unique self, but not to act egoistically, severing its relationship with the life of the body and failing to act in mutual synthesis with it.

The Peckham Biologists had a biological world-view, which is not at all the same as a 'scientific world-view', for the latter usually signifies a belief that the Earth and the life upon it obeys only the laws of physics and chemistry. They had a quite unsentimental reverence for nature and, therefore, a respect for the natural powers and needs of human beings. As physicians, they respected the power of the body to maintain its wholeness – to heal itself – and to regulate the behaviour of its parts for its own good, always provided that its external environment and food are suitable and the person's behaviour and state of mind are appropriate. It seemed to them likely that human beings are potentially as capable of acting for the good of the whole of which they are dependent parts as is a cell in a body, or a more simple organism in its ecosystem (its local bit of the biosphere). They saw that, because he is a social being, an individual human needs to be a part of a social whole with which he can be in a relationship of mutual synthesis and, if he is to maintain this whole, he must have an 'autonomous' relationship with it. He must have

* 1943, p. 25

an awareness of – a feeling for – it's needs, and act accordingly, whether this whole is biological or social – his family, the total biosphere, or a local neighbourhood community. Being an autonomous part of a whole means being oneself – acting spontaneously according to one's needs as a whole but also according to the needs of the greater whole of which one is a part. It means assuming responsibility for the whole. It was seen that the children at the Centre and in my playgroup assumed responsibility for the wholes that were the play situations of which they were free and spontaneously creative parts. (More of this below.)

In parentheses, at this point, I would like to consider a criticism that has been made to me of Scott Williamson's concept of a healthy person as one who is growing – developing his potential capacities to the full. It is suggested that a person who is doing this would also be developing his capacity to do evil. There is no doubt that this is true in the sense that, if evil is one's intention, greater skill and ability will increase one's ability to achieve it, but greater capability does not in itself increase the wish to do evil; therefore, in another sense, a person who has developed his potential powers to the full is no more capable of doing evil than he would have been if his powers had remained undeveloped. To anyone who knew the Centre well, it was evident that the members, young and old, were increasing their capability in many ways, and it was observed that their behaviour was, on the whole, the reverse of anti-social or egoistical. It was in the main expressive of a sense of responsibility for the club as a whole, and of a feeling for the value of others. Most of the time, most of the members chose to act in a way that was beneficial to their fellow-members and to the Centre as an institution. The children did the same to a quite astonishing extent.

It was observed that the relationship of individuals to their families had often a similarly 'autonomous' quality. This became apparent in some of the families who had, on joining, been composed of egoistically irresponsible or warring individuals. Membership of the Centre appeared to have the effect of enabling people to be active and creative parts of wholes that they valued. These wholes might be their own families, groups of friends, groups formed in order to pursue particular activities, or the society of the Centre as a whole. They behaved 'autonomously' in relation to these wholes; they acted in a way that benefited them – with responsibility for them.

I have noticed a surprising absence of the word 'responsibility' in the Peckham Biologists' later writing. Perhaps they avoided the use of the word because of its moral connotations, for they did not think of responsibility as a moral duty. To them it was a characteristic of health. In 1931 they wrote:

Responsibility implies the delicate poise of an organism about its own centre whilst versatile articulate relationships are maintained with each item of the environment... Responsibility is a biological attribute of consciousness; it is of the very essence of health.*

Summing up what has been said so far in this chapter, it seems to me that what happened at the Pioneer Health Centre is indicative of the truth of the following statements:

1) The freedom of action of a person who is a part of a whole on which he is dependent for existence, growth or happiness is limited. It is limited by his need to maintain the whole.

2) However richly diverse an environment may be, a person cannot be in a growth-promoting relationship of mutual synthesis with it, if it is beyond his power to make himself well acquainted with it, or if it changes substantially and frequently. If diversity is to be made use of, it must be digestible.

So, one has to say to Mill and von Humboldt that infinite diversity of surroundings plus freedom from all constraints will not by themselves produce a situation in which a person may achieve 'the highest and most harmonious development of his powers to a complete and consistent whole'. This ideal situation is more likely to occur when a person is a self-directing part of a greater social whole which he values and when his relation to this whole is autonomous in the 'Peckham' meaning of the word.

* * * * *

Twentieth-century conditions of life do not often allow people to be autonomous parts of a social whole in the Peckham sense. In the Stone Age however it may have been the usual way of life. Judging from our knowledge of the various peoples who still live mainly by hunting and gathering, in the same way as their (and our) ancestors did for hundreds of thousands of years, Stone Age people had certain advantages over twentieth-century urban peoples. The ecologist and anthropologist, Stephen Boyden has made a study of all the available literature on hunter-gatherer societies and has compiled a list of the likely health and happiness promoting life conditions (or 'the biological determinants of optimal health') of typical hunter-gatherer peoples. About half of these are physical conditions such as clean air and water and a healthy diet.†
The rest are what he calls 'intangible' conditions:

Close intimate relationship between infants and their mothers from the moment of birth; considerable 'community interaction' and exercise of responsibility towards other members of the community; co-operative

---

* 1931, p. 65

† Robert Milnes Coates says that recent research shows that even the Bushman living in near desert and the Eskimo have a balanced and varied diet containing all the various nutrients needed by man as long as they follow their traditional eating habits. 'What is a Natural Diet?' in *Nutrition and Health*, Vol. 1, No. 1.

small group interaction; incentives and opportunity for creative behaviour and the practice of learned manual skills; emphasis on active (e.g. dancing, singing, music making) rather than passive entertainment; short-term goal-achievement cycles (i.e. goals set and achieved usually in 24 hours or less); an environment which was full of interest; considerable variety in daily experience.

On the level of the biopsychic state, I suggest that it is reasonable to suspect that hunter-gatherers usually experienced a sense of personal involvement, a sense of purpose, a sense of belonging, a sense of interest in their surroundings and in their activities, a sense of comradeship, a sense of challenge and a sense of identity, and that their aspirations were of a kind likely to be fulfilled.*

It is probable that one of the most advantageous life conditions experienced by such peoples is that they live in smallish communities, ranging from families of half a dozen people to hunting 'bands' of not more than 100, including children. Each member of the group is aware that his welfare is dependent on the continued existence of the group, on its effectiveness in finding food and shelter and on the joyfulness and harmony of the relationships of its members.

Many of the small groups of people still living as they have always lived by hunting and gathering (or, as Richard Leakey insists, by 'gathering and hunting' since their basic everyday food is the leaves, seeds, fruit, roots and insects they collect and gather) have been driven into desert areas and are finding it more and more difficult to find enough of their previously health-promoting food and to retain their ancient culture and customs intact.

However, such tropical rain forests as remain still provide a healthy home for some the the peoples who have lived there possibly since Homo Sapiens evolved fully. The Mbuti Pygmies of the Ituri Forest are an example of a people whose essentially civilised social relationships and happy cohesiveness, combined with a great individual variety of personality and the custom of expressing their individuality spontaneously and vigorously are seemingly the result of the practice of autonomy in the Peckham sense.†

I use the present tense because I hope that they still follow the life described by Colin Turnbull nearly thirty years ago.¶

Hunting, for these Pygmies, is a communal activity; the game is driven by beaters (the women and older children) into a large semicircle of nets joined together and manned by marksmen armed with spears and bows and arrows. The method of hunting determines the size of the 'band'. The minimum is about seven families and a band rarely exceeds eighty people including children. From Turnbull's account, it seems that they have perfected the art of communal living. They have no chiefs, judges, priests, formal councils or laws, and almost no crime. There is a

* Boyden, 1980
† See Chapter 9 above for an account of their child-rearing paractices
¶ 1961

great deal of public discussion in which anyone may join. The elderly, some of whom are respected for their wisdom and looked up to, usually value tradition and encourage its preservation. At the same time, there is a marked absence of uniformity of behaviour; they are a highly individualistic and idiosyncratic people with a diversity of talents, attitudes, tastes and opinions. One trait they have in common, according to Turnbull, is a 'dislike of personal authority' and they avoid assuming it. if possible.

There is a traditional division of occupation between the sexes, that of the women being the more necessary for the welfare of the band, and also a traditional equality. There seems to be, in fact, almost no domination of one person by another.

They live their lives within the sight or hearing of everyone, except when they seek the solitude of the forest, and they are outspoken in condemnation of anything they consider to be anti-social. This may spark off furious argument. As with many non-literate peoples, most of them are very articulate; speaking is a highly developed art, and enjoyed so much that an argument rarely degenerates into physical violence, or, alternatively, results in bottled up resentment. A plea by one of the more peace-loving among them that there is too much noise (meaning angry noises) and, as a last resort, a reminder that 'the forest does not like noise' usually has a calming effect. Anyone present may contribute an opinion, or the lessening of tension by tickling the Mbuti's strong sense of the ridiculous. If there is persistent anti-social behaviour, it may be dealt with by ostracism, the threat of which will often bring the offender to heel. Lasting antagonisms may be resolved by the decision of an individual or a family to join another band. There is not infrequent visiting of relatives between bands, but the possibility of transfer to another band will depend on whether or not it is already at the optimum size for hunting. An awareness of their need for the band contributes to the preservation of an overall harmony and a spontaneous co-operation among these lively, laughter-loving and independent-minded people.

It is interesting that their respect for their fellows does not extend to non-pygmies. They do not consider the agriculturalists of a different race who live on the edge of the forest to be fully human – 'those others are animals!' – and will, on occasion, cheat them and steal food from their fields when they can safely do so. They use their story-telling and descriptive talents to increase the superstitious fear that these outsiders have of the forest.

When a much admired or loved person dies, the band holds a 'Molimo' festival which continues for two or three to twenty evenings and well into the night. There is singing and sometimes dancing. The songs are songs of thanksgiving for the life of the deceased and of praise for the forest. The Mbuti also sing when there is a serious shortage of game or some other disaster. Then they sing to awaken the forest, which seems to them to have been temporarily asleep and neglectful of their needs. 'We wake it up by our singing and we do this because we want it to awaken happy. We sing to rejoice the Forest.'

Like the Australian Aboriginals, who say – or have said – 'The land does not belong to us: we belong to the land,' the Pygmies feel that they are part of the forest – children of the forest. They know that they are entirely dependent on it for their well-being and that it provides for them well and abundantly; and they are grateful. They study its secrets and respect its' needs. They live in an 'autonomous' relationship with it, in which a process of mutual synthesis between individual and environment takes place. For example, each hunting band has it's own hunting area within which it moves around in order not to destroy the food sources within any part of it.

It is clear that there is much to learn from the Mbuti. We could begin by giving our children an example of a similar degree of reverence for our world as the Pygmies do to theirs. To them, the forest is the world. Our world consists of the whole of the surface of the Earth. So our task, the task of preserving and cultivating it's health (and consequently our own as well) is very much more complicated than theirs but, it is to be hoped, not impossible.

Since Colin Turnbull learned to love and respect the Mbuti Pygmies, anthropologists have discovered that they are by no means a unique phenomenon. In her introduction to *Politics and History in Band Societies* (1982) which she edited with Richard Lee, Eleanor Leacock wrote:

> In our view, there is a core of features common to band-living foraging societies around the world ... Similarities include egalitarian patterns of sharing; strong anti-authoritarianism; an emphasis on the importance of co-operation together with great respect for individuality; marked flexibility in band membership and in living arrangements generally; permissive child-rearing practices; and common techniques for handling problems of conflict and reinforcing group cohesion such as teasing and joking, endless talking and the ritualization of potential antagonisms.

There is evidence to show that foraging people have lived for many centuries in contact with farming communities. For example, the Mbuti Pygmies have lost their original language and speak a dialect of one or other of the agricultural peoples who live on the outskirts of the forest, but they have preserved intact their own way of life and beliefs.

The suggestion has been made that these primitive peoples have, at birth, neither more nor less of a tendency to be aggressive, competitive, envious, or generous than so-called civilised peoples, and that it is the effect of the kind of social environment and the wise upbringing that they have experienced that makes the majority of them independent-minded and capable individuals and, at the same time, spontaneously co-operative and responsible members of a group.

It is good to learn that some peoples such as the Australian Aborigine, the Eskimo and the Indians of the Arctic have, during the last fifteen years or so, begun to halt the trend towards their absorption into industrialised society by learning how to fight successfully for their right to wander, hunt and gather over certain areas, in courts of law. Forest-dwelling foragers are, however, dependent for survival on the continued presence of forests.

* * * * *

As we have seen, the Centre members, old and young, were able to be 'autonomous' and, therefore, responsible parts of wholes which they valued. What was it that made them capable of sustaining these wholes? How was it that they were aware of the needs of the wholes, both in the long term and from moment to moment, so that they were able to exercise responsibility for them?

I hope I shall be forgiven for once again reverting to the simple situations that occurred in my free-choice playgroup, for an illustration of the point I want to make in an attempt to answer this question. In my playgroup, at any moment, the whole of which the children were parts was the total ever-changing play situation, but at the same time it might also be a smaller play situation within the total, perhaps a transitory game of 'Mothers and Fathers' engaged in by two or three children. Watching these games, one could see a child changing his behaviour and adapting it to what he perceived would fit in with another child's desires and intentions, in order that the game might continue. For the children soon became aware that with so many attractive alternative pursuits close at hand, a 'mother', for example, could very easily lose her 'baby' or a 'baby' her 'mother'. Because they valued these wholes (the games they were creating) the children did their best to maintain them, and so they made themselves responsible for the smooth running of the game. They wanted to maintain these wholes, but they were also such as they were able to maintain. The reasons for this were, I believe, firstly, that they were limited in extent, and, secondly, that each child usually knew his playmates well and, even if he did not, had a sympathy with and an understanding of the needs of the others in relation to the game being played; so he was capable of responding appropriately to the whole situation.

It was the same with the rather older children in the Centre gymnasium. There, as we have seen, the material surroundings and the activity were entirely of a kind with which the children were familiar or could easily make themselves familiar, and were contained within a space small enough to allow the children to be aware through their senses of the situation within the whole at any moment.

To some extent, the situation was similar in the whole that was the Centre. Owing mainly to the design of the building, the members were easily able to make themselves acquainted with the potentialities for activity that the building offered, with what went on in the various groups and intra-mural clubs, and with the other members, old and young. The activity of each was visible to all, and opportunities for informal encounters plentiful. As we have seen, people came to know each other very well through exercising their talents and abilities together – often for a common end, through learning from and helping each other as members of the various clubs, through the friendships and activities of their children and the advent of new babies. For most of its existence, the Centre had an active membership of more than 500 families (1,800 to 2,000 individuals); therefore nobody could know all the other members personally, but each could get to know a large number of them well. Like the children in my playgroup, the members could feel at home in the Centre; they could feel confident of acting appropriately to the needs of the situation because, although the environment was diverse, it was stable. It did not change violently or incomprehensibly; there were no sudden changes imposed from above or instituted by a committee of members on a majority decision. Instead, people's environment within the Centre grew or evolved from innumerable small initiatives and inter-actions and from the growth of people's individualities. It was continually diversifying, little by little, but the changes were easily assimilable by the individual, who could maintain his familiarity with it. Regarding the situation within the smaller whole of the family, it was evident to us that people got to know and understand their own family members better, as they observed them responding to the larger and more diverse environment of the Centre, and this made an individual increasingly capable of 'autonomy' towards his or her family.

One might think that very young children would only be capable of acting autonomously in relation to a very small group. It is therefore interesting to observe that when children under five are in an environment that is suitable for play and where they are free of unnecessary interference by their elders, they will choose to play individually or in small groups of two or three, but will continuously act in awareness of the larger whole, and that this ability for awareness of the situation can extend to quite a large group. One day I sat and watched for an hour in a playgroup consisting of 45 children all together in one large hall. This was an unusually large number for a pre-school playgroup, but the group was, in my view, exceptionally happy and successful. The material environment was organised extremely well: equipment, apparatus and toys were set out so that the children could use what they wanted, when and how they wanted, and no organisation of the children was necessary. Each child knew he was responsible for himself and his enjoyment, and acted accordingly. Since the spontaneous movement of the children, some running and jumping, some on tricycles or pushing dolls' prams and trolleys in between the tables, box of dressing-up clothes, group of painting easels, and the slide and climbing frame, at all of which children were playing, did not result (while I was watching) in collisions or quarrels, it is to be concluded that each child was as much aware of all this activity as was necessary if he was to be able to fit his purposes into what was going on in the hall as a whole. If children of three or four years of age can behave like this, there are grounds for hope in a future for mankind.

Like most faculties, the faculty for responsibility needs to be exercised if it is to develop. As we have seen, a baby who is consistently in a situation that favours human growth, exercises responsibility for his own growth, for the development of his faculties including the 'faculty for choice'. The growth of the latter enables him to be increasingly capable of exercising responsibility for himself and his surroundings. But this can only happen if, for some part of every day, children are allowed to choose, and to face the consequences. If, on the other hand, they know that someone is *always* hovering, ready to put things straight for them whenever they make a misjudgement or things go wrong, or to smooth out quarrels – ready, in fact, to usurp their responsibility, so that they have no need to look where they are going or to be aware of what is happening around them – they cannot learn to take the responsibility for their own safety and enjoyment nor to take a responsible part in maintaining and initiating enjoyable play situations; they cannot learn to be responsible for their environment. One observes that some adults take on themselves more than their fair share of responsibility for others and for the environment generally, while others appear to be incapable of being responsible even for their own welfare and are willing to leave this to others. Now and again there is a child who seems to have an inherent tendency to abdicate the responsibility for his safety and amusement in favour of his parents or others, if they are anxious to take it over. No doubt, a child's behaviour in this respect – as in others – is the result of the effect of the interaction of his inherent characteristics and his environmental situation. But, if children do not have the opportunity to be responsible even for amusing and entertaining themselves, it must surely be difficult for them to develop any potentiality they may have for the faculty to be responsible for themselves and their surroundings – to develop this biological characteristic of health.

* * * * *

I believe that by the end of the third year of the main experiment, the Peckham Biologists already felt that they had an answer to their question, 'What is the nature of health?' At the Centre, as we have seen, at any time a child or an adult could be – and most were – a spontaneously acting and 'autonomous' part of several social wholes, and, with each whole, he could be – and often was – in a relationship of mutual synthesis. The Biologists saw this happening. They saw what they understood to be health developing. They felt that circumstances had been created within which some, at least, of the biological laws governing the health of human organisms could operate. They wrote:

> In the coming years, we are all going to discover that we must either learn to understand and live in obedience to the laws of biology, thereby coming to live more abundantly; or that by ignoring them our misfortunes must multiply till, heaping up, they ultimately destroy man's civilisation – and even man himself.*

They felt that they had contributed to our knowledge of these laws. The next problem was how to communicate their findings to others. Scott Williamson's main purpose during the last years of his life was to devise scientifically objective terms in which to embody his findings.

Scott Williamson did not formalise these laws, but he defined health as 'a progressive mutual synthesis participated in by both organism and environment'. From this it follows that an organism needs to be in a relationship of mutual synthesis with its environment if it is to flourish. This means, as we have seen, that it needs to be a part of a whole, a progressively familiar but diverse and growing whole (or wholes), and to act as a whole itself – not as a mass of unconnected or warring parts.

Another biological law that an organism must obey – or perhaps one should rather say, another condition that is necessary for its health, another biological need – is the opportunity to realise its unique individuality, which is one of the qualities that distingushes an organism from a thing – or an unhealthy organism.

A third need is the opportunity to grow, by means of the subjective synthesis of elements or experiences of its environment, according to its potentiality. For this, it needs to be able to take the physical, mental and emotional nourishment that is appropriate to its specific growth needs at that moment.

Fourthly, it needs the opportunity to exercise and develop another characteristic of organisms: the power to choose the precise bit of 'nourishment' it needs at a particular moment in time. Its choice is influenced not only by its own needs but also by its awareness of the needs of the various wholes of which it is a part.

Most of the long-term members of the Centre we have contacted are aware that it provided them with an opportunity to grow and to enjoy life that they had not had before, and that the effect on them of the years during which they made the Centre a part of their lives and themselves a part of the Centre had proved lasting. Visitors commented on the 'atmos-

* 1943

phere' emanating from the happy interactions between the members. In this book, I have quoted some members' and one or two visitors' attempts to describe precisely what they experienced. I have also tried to convey, in simple language, the understanding of what was happening in the Centre that my later experiences and, during the last 20 years, a preoccupation with 'Peckham' theory, have given me. It seems to me that ordinary English should be adequate because we are organisms; we experience health – and the lack of it; we are able to observe it in babies and animals; we should be able to understand the laws that govern the health of our own biological nature when they are described in the kind of words which we use to describe our own feelings and experiences.

The physicist and astronomer, Fred Hoyle, once remarked that the laws of physics are simple but the effects of the operation of these laws are of infinite variety and complexity. It seems to me that this is even more applicable in the field of biology. The organisms that are the products of the operation of simple and universal biological laws are so various and so extremely complex that it is possibly beyond the power of the human intellect to follow accurately their functioning and their inter-actions with each other. Recent discoveries of the body's bio-chemical make up and needs are an example of this complexity and of the hereto unimagined subtlety of the balance of the nutrients it needs in order to function healthily. This being the case, it seems to me to be important to wonder whether health – in ourselves and others, in social institutions and events and in nature – is something that may be appreciable only by the individual person, exercising his awareness as a whole. It is probable that it cannot be assessed satisfactorily or defined accurately either mathematically or verbally. Perhaps, like love, beauty or terror, it is an experience that can best be communicated to others by the use of meta-phor or poetic imagery. Certainly its existence cannot be proved or disproved. So, we must have more faith in our personal awareness and judgement, and have a greater respect for what the scientist and philoso-pher, Michael Polanyi, has called 'tacit knowing'.

At the close of a recent unsigned but, in general, perceptive and appreciative article in *The Lancet*, it was implied that Scott Williamson and Innes Pearse had failed to prove what they set out to prove, which was that 'the study and cultivation of health would diminish the incidence of disease and the cost of health care.' I do not believe that it was their intention to prove this. Moreover, it seems to me, particularly in view of the fact that it is the degenerative diseases we are most likely to succumb to today, including the loss of the body's ability to dis-tinguish correctly between – and behave appropriately towards – poten-tial friend and potential foe, that no rational person would require proof of the proposition that the study and cultivation of positive health would diminish the incidence of disease. We must take care that we do not allow the habit we have acquired of suspending action until proof of its value has been set out on paper, to cause us to lose the ability to use our reason.

However, the Peckham Biologists' hypothesis is discoverable in their writings, especially in the best-seller of 45 years ago, *The Peckham Experiment*. People were impressed by the originality and wisdom of this book. To me their hypothesis is plain common sense. It is this that I find so exciting because it causes me to feel that it must contain accurate reflections of the truth. This may sound arrogant but, since natural selection would have seen to it that our earliest human ancestors obeyed the biological laws that govern health in humans, it is understandable that, when these laws are pointed out to us, they should appear to be common sense.

I hope that the contents of this book will appeal to other people's common sense too.

I hope that it will stimulate people to look at the world and everything in it from a biological point of view, and I hope also that it will incline students of biology (the science of life) to think about the basic nature of life as well as about the one specialised form or microscopic bit of it that they have chosen to work upon.

Chapter 12

Today and Tomorrow

People say, 'A Peckham Centre would never succeed today – society is too sick.' They instance the vandalism and mindless violence, the apparent decline of the family, and the time spent watching television. They may add that the failure to find paid employment and the enforced dependence for a livelihood on others erodes the sense of self-worth that is essential to health, and that the search for jobs or advancement causes a mobility that destroys the chances of creating stable communities. It is certainly true that, in many ways, social conditions have become more detrimental to health during the last 40 years, yet it is also true that the intellectual climate is now much more favourable for the understanding and acceptance of the value of the Peckham Biologists' work and ideas. The increasingly obvious pollution and unsuitability for health of the environment that we as a civilisation are making for ourselves and for wildlife is causing more people to question the value of our commercially subservient lifestyle, to doubt the wisdom of blindly riding roughshod over nature, and to do what they can to stop or repair the damage. More people are open to the value of Scott Williamson's insights and able to understand his thought because *their* thoughts have begun to travel along similar paths.

An example of this is a growing humility in scientists studying the chemistry and nutritional needs of the human body when they find that its complexity defeats understanding, and that to interfere with the subtle balance of its functioning is only too easy and very dangerous.

An example of the practical effects that the recognition of the wholeness, the unity, of a living being is having is the research being undertaken into the relationship of nutrition and behaviour, and also nutrition and schizophrenia and other psychological maladies.

In his 1978 James Mackenzie Memorial Lecture, Dr W W Yellowlees gave the Royal College of General Practitioners both hope and an urgent warning and call to action. After contrasting the usual diet during the twentieth century of the people of his practice in the Highlands of Scotland with the much healthier one in previous centuries, he said:

> The new epidemics of degenerative disease are not inevitable, nor is their cause mysterious. They are nature's language, telling eloquently of our failure to understand the supreme importance of nature's laws.

Had he been alive in 1978, Scott Williamson would certainly have expressed a similar view.

There are obstetricians such as Michel Odent and many midwives who are working to provide women with the chance to co-operate with nature in giving birth and nurturing the baby, and to spare them unnecessary technological interference in what can be the most satisfying and exhilarating experience of a lifetime.*

Without any help from governments, individual organic farmers and market gardeners are tenaciously working to restore and maintain the viability and vitality of the fields and meadows they tend and to produce food that will sustain the vitality and resistance to disease of people – food that contains the full variety of nutrients needed by human beings and does not contain chemicals that the human body cannot tolerate. They must be satisfying a demand because most of them are making a living.

Among scientists and philosophers there are voices to be heard calling for recognition of the instinctive wisdom of wildlife and of 'hunter-gatherer' peoples that live in what is in fact a relationship of mutual synthesis with their particular areas of the biospere. And there are some who call passionately to mankind to preserve – for their sanity's sake – the wilderness, to save areas of untamed nature, as well as managed open spaces, so that people may enhance their joy-in-life and strengthen their will-to-live through the sight and sound and touch and smell of nature, as their forbears were able to do throughout the evolution of our species up to now.

Until his death in 1986, hundreds of families and individuals camped in a sometimes muddy field in Hampshire during the month of September, to listen to J Krishnamurti telling them that they must rid themselves of the conditioning that everyone acquires (even thinking, he said, tends to be a mechanical activity that runs in habitual grooves); they must stop criticising and judging and only 'observe', with mind and senses open to as much as possible of the whole of their surroundings, near and far, and then act with spontaneity. As the reader will be aware, this is very close to Scott Williamson's thinking.

But it is not only a few pioneers in their professions who are displaying a new reverence for life and a desire to learn the true nature and essential needs of the human organism. The change is also a grass-roots phenomenon. People whose thoughts and actions no-one ever reads about are allowing their biological wisdom to surface. They no longer assume that the accepted intellectual, political and religious leaders of society will be wiser and better informed than themselves; they are paying attention to their own instincts and trusting their own judgement. This is especially true of parents seeking health-enhancing conditions of life for their children, for they begin to wonder what sort of life will be possible in 30 years' time. They are wanting to change the direction in

* Odent, 1976, 1978, 1989

which humankind is moving. They want to create an environment in which their children may become capable of thinking for themselves and also of *being* their real selves, and in which they may learn how to relate sensitively and responsibly to others and to be creative parts of lasting social wholes. Such independent minds tend to value opportunities for rich personal relationships above material riches, to value growth in the quality of life above growth in the GNP and to put the positive, holistic health of people the world over first of all.

However it is still often difficult to get one's meaning across to others on the subject of health, because the habit of misusing the word is so ingrained. The word 'health' is so often used to mean its opposite – sickness – that it tends to be associated in people's minds with the care of ill-health, with remedial and therapeutic institutions and personnel. This, I think, can be the only explanation for a doctor of medicine, who claimed to be in favour of setting up Peckham-type centres, saying that the Peckham researchers were concerned with health and therefore could not have discovered anything relevant to the theory and practice of education.

That health is something positive, something more than the absence of disease and disability has always been instinctively known: the 'blooming cheek', 'clear eye', 'shining hair' or 'springing step'. Now, nearly half a century after the Peckham Biologists demonstrated this truth in an experimental situation, and tried to make it accepted as a fact by the established leaders of thought and makers of policy, it is at last seeping into people's conscious thoughts, and they are beginning to ponder its implications.

An understanding and acceptance of the idea, put forward by the Peckham Biologists, that *health is basically a process of realising one's potential for maturity* would make communication on the subject of health easier and the practice of education healthier.

If health is a process of mutual subjective synthesis of organism and environment and of person and group, it is not something that members of the medical profession can give us. They can only remove or alleviate the pathological conditions that prevent us from engaging in the process of health. The responsibility for a person's health lies firstly with himself and, secondly, with anyone who has any power to influence his environment, lawmakers, administrators, planners, architects, teachers, farmers, processors of foodstuffs – and parents.

Local and national government services have difficulty in providing the resources and personnel necessary to deal with all the sickness and incapacity in the population. As a body, they cannot look beyond this, and only a very few of the overworked individuals so employed have the energy to make time to think on the subject of health and how best to promote it. Therefore I believe that people will have to make up their own minds individually what they want in the way of the means of cultivating health, find out how it may be obtained, and go out and get it for themselves.

As I have suggested, it is probably the parents of young children more than any other class of people who are strongly moved to create for themselves an environment in which health may be cultivated. It seems to me that many of them feel that the purpose of life is life and that their prime responsibility is to the next generation. And some have a similar confidence to that which developed in the Peckham Centre, in the capacity for spontaneous growth of every living being, in a person's inborn urge to grow, and in his power to recognise the particular nourishment that his faculties and abilities need at any moment in order to grow, as long as his environment contains suitable opportunities for nourishment. Many among them also know that it does not help children to have parents who feel that they must sacrifice their own growth for the children's sake. They know – as the Peckham Biologists knew – that the best surroundings for a child are such as contain people who are rejoicing in their own growth and who enjoy doing whatever they are doing at the moment (including the household chores and whatever else is necessary for the creation of a home that gives pleasure and allows the family individuality to develop).

Tragedies and disasters make the news, and this may mislead us into thinking that the family as a social institution is dead. In fact it is very much alive. Even the marriage ceremony is not by any means a dying tradition, followed only by those who are members of churches or wish to please their elderly relations. There are couples, unorthodox and unconventional in every way, who choose to plight their troth and exchange rings before an official of church or state and a gathering of their friends, relatives and neighbours because they wish to make public their intention to form a stable biological unit and to become a creative part of a personal community of known and loved people.

It seems that people who are trying to make for their children a more health-enhancing environment – including more community life – are experiencing a need to live among others of like mind. They are finding it difficult to lead a life that is different from their neighbours and, at the same time, be a part of a neighbourhood community. They find it hard to enable their children to develop their faculty to be self-directing and responsible when their neighbours' children are not enabled so to do. It is difficult for children to exercise their faculty for choice when their surroundings do not contain appropriate growth-promoting experiences or opportunities for action from which to choose. How, for example, does one prevent children from becoming accustomed to heavily salted or sweetened foods – ice lollies and crisps or caffeine-containing coca-cola, from expecting ready-made entertainment and the latest expensive science-fiction type toy, or from acting in a more violent, destructive and anti-social manner than they would naturally do, if this is the usual behaviour of their playmates. It is difficult for couples to go it alone without either losing their children's confidence or inculcating in them a 'holier than thou' attitude to others.

A young family of my acquaintance in Tucson, Arizona, have begun to form a 'network' of families – calling itself *Making Contact* – who share their longing to live among people with similar values and aims. They have been encouraged in their efforts by discovering the work of the Peckham Biologists. Their intention is to get to know each other through correspondence with a view to moving house eventually to some agreed location. They are naturally impatient to make a start with the formation of a more growth-promoting environment for themselves and their children and they believe that even a small group of 15 to 20 families, if they had sufficient values in common, could make a beginning of a rewarding community life. They do *not* propose a commune with pooling of incomes and shared accommodation: they realise the importance of a private 'territory' for each family. They envisage the families living as near together as possible and owning in common a building of some kind which could be used as a community centre. A venture as small as this would not be a Pioneer Health Centre, but, if the members of the group were convinced of the truth and value of the biological principles on which the Centre was based and were dedicated to finding a way to implement them, it might be a seed from which one could grow.

Innes Pearse held that a piecemeal method of attack would be unsuccessful, and that if any of the beneficial effects of the Peckham Centre are to be achieved, it will be necessary to recreate the whole, the complex and comprehensive whole. I have an uncomfortable feeling that she may be right. Yet there is no doubt that Peckham-type centres will be different is some ways from the prototype; people's basic needs do not change but their circumstances have changed; (these include available knowledge of the body's nutritional needs). Centres will, also, be different from each other; for example, city dwellers' needs are slightly different from those of the inhabitants of rural areas. It is certain that in the cold and temperate zones of the world a building in which to meet will be necessary: the town square or the village green is not good enough. As we have seen, the building designed by Scott Williamson was ideal as a base for a social community. It is to be hoped that it will not remain only an ideal. For what it offered, it was relatively inexpensive to build; a luxury cinema of the period cost five times as much. It is however an inescapable fact that considerable financial resources would have to be available to a group of people if they were to build premises of a similar kind. Moreover, the Peckham building was expensive to run, with its swimming pool and its partially glass walls, but it may be that the running costs could be considerably reduced by the use of modern techniques and materials.

In my view, a group of families devoted to the Peckham philosophy would be likely to seek certain minimum conditions for the cultivation of health:

1) A building as near as resources permit to the original design.
2) A subscription-paying and local family membership of the Centre.
3) Access to whole, organically grown foodstuffs and the opportunity to grow some of them locally.
4) Opportunity to obtain pre-conception (for both parents), ante-natal and post-natal *health* overhauls.
5) Access to a health-orientated baby clinic, extended to include health overhauls – at less frequent intervals – for older children.
6) The opportunity to live near enough to the building for the children of the member-families to use it individually and in their own time.

The children should be able to come and go on their own, to come even if they have only an hour to spare or to stay for the whole of Saturday afternoon. If they were to be obliged to wait until their parents could take them by car, or escort them by public transport, or to be dependent on the prearranged escort of family friends, they would not be able to use the building in the way the Centre was used by the Peckham children, and which proved to be so conducive to their healthy growth and development, and to the development of the all-age community that was one of the Centre's unique features. A weekly visit is likely to be only frustrating to a young child (and a frustrated child is an unhappy child, often an antisocial child). He may be longing to take his skill a stage further and, after a week with no chance to do so, finds his body has 'forgotten' the skill he already had. Too much of this can weaken a child's confidence in his power to learn what he wants to learn.

Aside from this, it is surely important that children should be enabled to gain the pleasure and self-respect that making their *own* way to a playspace, swimming pool, library or school can give them. It cannot add to one's self-esteem or to the growth of one's power of responsibility or of one's ability to respond appropriately, realistically and wisely to circumstances to be *taken* everywhere as if one were a baby or a parcel.

As we have seen, the Peckham Experiment provided evidence of the kind of physical and social circumstances that enable people – children and adults – to develop their mental, physical and social faculties and talents to their own satisfaction. Perhaps the most important of these circumstances was the opportunity to be freely functioning parts of wholes greater than themselves with which they could be in a relationship of mutual synthesis. One way of envisaging the process of growth through mutual synthesis is as a spiral:

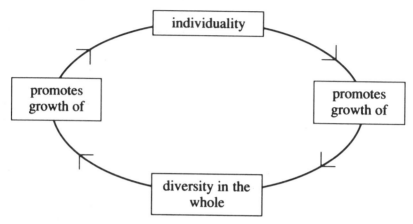

This crude diagram does not show all the necessary conditions that enable the process of mutual synthesis to happen – of which, as we have seen, one of the most important is the familiarity of the individual with the physical and social whole of which he is a part.

In the environment that evolved at the Peckham Centre, the spiral of healthy growth operated. How can such an environment be recreated? How can we best use the knowledge gained at Peckham? In my view, only by thoroughly digesting it and making it our own, and then getting together with others who have chosen to do the same, and selecting such of the circumstances that obtained at the Peckham Centre that we, as a group, most want, and proceeding to create them for ourselves.

I feel that at the stage civilisation has reached in industrialised countries, a group – that is, a family or a larger social unit such as a local community – can only create the conditions within itself in which health can flourish if the individuals composing it have some awareness of the fundamental nature of human growth-needs. People may be aware of these needs in different ways, intellectually, intuitively or through being sensitive to their own experience. I believe that a study of the PHC literature can help people of all types to become conscious of their understanding of these needs and, therefore, more capable of creating for themselves, in co-operation with others, the kind of health-promoting social and physical conditions that were created by the biologists and the member-families of the Pioneer Health Centre in St Mary's Road, Peckham.

The Peckham Biologists were successful in producing a situation in which a stable and health-promoting community could grow because, firstly, their hypothesis of the nature of health and of the conditions in which it can flourish turned out to be largely correct and, as good scientists, they modified it when necessary in the light of the facts that emerged during the course of the experiment. Secondly, the members joined on the understanding that they were taking part in an experiment and must, therefore, accept the final authority of the directors of the experiment. For example, although the members were expected to initiate and organise activities for themselves, there was a limitation on their freedom to organise or direct each other, and a definite ban on the institution of an elected central committee; for the latter would, the Biologists feared, have meant the direction, by a few leader-type members, of the rest, and the inhibiting of the growth of 'autonomy'. Perhaps, in time, an understanding of the needs of health would have spread to all – or a sufficient majority of – the members so that the Biologists would no longer have had any need to act in order to safeguard the freedom, spontaneity and responsibility of the individual. There were signs that this could happen. As we have seen, most of the members had a strong feeling of responsibility towards the whole, and many appreciated the potential value to the whole of the contribution of each individual. But, I fear that to set up a new Centre on Peckham lines – without any watchful team containing a Scott Williamson, an Innes Pearse and a Lucy Crocker to run it – in any existing populated area, with the expectation that people would use it in the same manner as the Peckham families after a year or so of membership had become accustomed to do, would be to invite failure.

The point I am trying to make is that it will be necessary to begin with the people rather than with the bricks and mortar, to begin by forming groups of families who are enthusiastic for the idea of creating a Centre on 'Peckham' lines *for their own use*. These families will have to be sufficiently convinced of the value of the discoveries made at Peckham concerning health – the health of individuals, families and communities – to be willing, if necessary, to move to the neighbourhood chosen by the group as a whole. They would also need to be willing to contribute financially according to their ability and according to the value they put on health, in addition to a minimum membership subscription. Perhaps, when the worth of Peckham-type Centres has been demonstrated several times over, public money may become available, as it is at present to the sports and leisure centres already built all over the country. In the meantime, it will be necessary to exercise a truly pioneering spirit. It may happen that a strong organising committee is needed to push such a project forward to opening day. If so, on that day, they will have to have the self-control to dissolve themselves, so that members and community can be free to grow through mutual synthesis.*

Perhaps it would be possible for such a pioneering group to get in at the planning stage of a projected new housing development, and see to it

---

* See Chapter 3

that it contains dwellings of various sizes (and prices), schools (or at least one primary school), an area of land suitable for horticulture (allotments or a market garden), a space large enough for a Centre-type building and routes to this space from all sides that can be safely taken by unaccompanied children. It was this sort of plan that was envisaged by Dr Kenneth Barlow and the 350 families who joined the 'Family Health Club Housing Association' in Coventry.*

Judging both from my memories of the Centre and from the opinions expressed by former members I have contacted over the last few years, it was the community that evolved within the membership – the fellowship, the fun and the affection that the member-families enjoyed with each other – that was the most memorable and health and happiness promoting effect of the Centre. A community such as this, composed of autonomous people (in the Peckham sense of free and spontaneously relating individuals, acting with responsibilty for the whole) cannot be created to order or wished on people. It has to grow. At Peckham it grew in the soil prepared for it by Scott Williamson and his colleagues. In the future, it will be necessary for people who regard such a community as an ideally healthy environment to understand fully the nature of the conditions in which it can grow and to want to create and maintain such conditions *for themselves.* The writings of Scott Williamson, Innes Pearse and Lucy Crocker and the actions of the member-families of the Centre have shown the way. It is worthwhile studying both in detail.

To me, it seems indisputable that a similar community could grow, if the large majority of the membership of a Centre newly starting up were to have a strong faith in the human potential for health, and an understanding of the means whereby the members of the Peckham Centre began to realise this potential in themselves. Perhaps such people would tend to be unusually reflective types. But if, when the Centre had got going, the membership were to be gradually swelled by other families inhabiting the neighbourhood, the mixture of types and tastes necessary in order to provide sufficient diversity might soon be achieved.

Gratitude for the years of membership of the Peckham Centre is still, after nearly half a century, strongly felt by all the members we have contacted in recent years. An astonishing loyalty to the ideas on which the Centre was founded and which grew out of it is also felt by others who knew it well, and even by some who never saw it in operation and have learned of it only through the literature. This long-standing enthusiasm is evidence of a conviction that, if similar centres of community life were available to the inhabitants of towns and conurbations the world over, society would be healthier and people would be happier and more fulfilled, balanced and responsible.

In this chapter, I have mentioned some of the difficulties that might be encountered by anyone trying to duplicate the Pioneer Health Centre.

* See Chapter 6, p. 116

But we must be careful not to let these distract us from making quite sure that we have understood and assimilated the discoveries made in the Peckham Experiment. We must allow ourselves to fully explore and follow up their implications.

What lay behind the success of the Centre was the faith that Scott Williamson and Innes Pearse and their colleagues and an increasing number of the member-families had in people's capacity for health – for achieving wholeness, individuality and creativity through the exercise of mutual synthesis with their environment. It was this faith that was the rock on which the Centre was built. But more than this was necessary for the success of this experiment in the cultivation of health. What was necessary was an understanding of the biological needs of humans, a knowledge of the conditions that are necessary for health.

Many of us may find it impossible to create the circumstances in which a health-promoting community similar to the Centre can evolve, but if, in our work as parents, nursery teachers, play leaders, students of human development, and planners, legislators and administrators of every kind, we can keep the Peckham Biologists' discoveries firmly in mind, and so can work with nature instead of against her, we shall be on the right track. Among other things, we shall make it easier for the young to develop their faculty for 'autonomy' and as a result we may be instrumental in swelling to an effective majority the number of people who feel a responsibility for their environment and who realise that they are dependent for their health and happiness on the welfare of the whole biospere – on the health of the planet Earth. Is it too much to hope, I wonder, that fear of the deterioration of the health of our planet and its inhabitants might serve, just as well as fear of the proverbial invasion from Mars, to unite all nations and religions, and might cause all peoples to redirect their energy to the discovery of how to maintain the delicate balance of the Earth's biosphere and of all its parts for the sake of generations to come?

References and Bibliography

The Peckham Biologists

Pearse, Innes H, **1926**, 'Racial Culture', *The Journal of State Medicine*, Vol. 34, No. 10

Pearse, Innes H, and Williamson, G Scott **1931**, *The Case for Action*, Faber and Faber, reprinted by Scottish Academic Press (1985)

Williamson, G Scott and Pearse, Innes H, **1938**, *Biologists in Search of Material*, Faber and Faber, reprinted by Scottish Academic Press (1985)

Pearse, Innes H, and Crocker, Lucy H, **1943**, *The Peckham Experiment: a study of the living structure of society*, George Allen and Unwin, reprinted by Scottish Academic Press (1985)

Williamson, G Scott and Pearse, Innes H, **1965**, *Science, Synthesis and Sanity: an enquiry into the nature of living*, Collins, reprinted by Scottish Academic Press, (1986)

Pearse, Innes H, **1979**, *The Quality of Life: the Peckham approach to human ethology*, Scottish Academic Press

Barlow, Kenneth, **1988**, *Recognising Health*, Kenneth Barlow, 24 Paddington Street, London W1M 4DR

Other authors

Allport, Gordon, **1937**, *Pattern and Growth in Personality*, New York, Holt, Rinehardt and Winston

Ashton, John, **1977**, 'The Peckham Pioneer Health Centre: a reappraisal', *Community Health*, 8, 132

Axline, Virginia M, **1964**, *Dibbs in Search of Self*, Pelican Books, (1971)

Bettleheim, Bruno, **1967**, *The Empty Fortress: infantile autism and the birth of the self*, The Free Press, New York

Boyden, Stephen and Miller, Sheelagh, **1978**, 'Human Ecology and the Quality of Life', *Urban Ecology*, No. 3 (1978)

Boyden, Stephen, **1980**, 'The Need for an Holistic Approach to Human Health and Wellbeing', *Changing Disease Patterns and Human Behaviour*, Stanley, N F and Joske, R A (eds), The Academic Press

Boyden, Stephen, **1987**, *Western Civilisation in Biological Perspective: patterns in biohistory*. Oxford University Press

Bruner, J and Connolly, S (eds), **1972**, *The Growth of Competence*, The Academic Press

Comerford, John, **1947**, *Health the Unknown: the story of the Peckham Experiment*, Hamish Hamilton

Donner, Florinda, **1982**, *Shabono*, The Bodley Head and Triad/Paladin (1984)

Fossey, Diane, **1984**, *Gorillas in the Mist*, Mowat; new edition, *Women in the Mist*, Macdonald (1988)

Goble, Frank, **1970**, *The Third Force*, Pocket Books, New York

Goodall, Jane, **1971**, *In the Shadow of Man*, Collins

Groos, Karl, **1901**, *The Play of Man*

Harlow, Harry F and Margaret K, **1962**, 'Social Deprivation in Monkeys', *Scientific American*, November 1962

Leacock, Eleanor and Lee, Richard, **1982**, *Politics and History in Band Societies*, Cambridge University Press

Liedloff, Jean, **1975**, *The Continuum Concept*, Gerald Duckworth; also Penguin Books (1986) and Addison-Wesley (1987)

Lovelock, J E, **1979**, *Gaia: a new look at life on earth*, Oxford University Press

Mansfield, Peter, **1988**, *Good Health Handbook*, Grafton

Maslow, Abraham H, **1968**, *Toward a Psychology of Being*, Van Nostrand

Mech, L D, **1966**, *The Wolves of Isle Royal*

Mech, L D, **1970**, *The Wolf: the ecology and behaviour of an endangered species*

Midgley, Mary, **1978**, *Beast and Man: the roots of human nature*, The Harvester Press (1979) and Methuen (1980)

Mill, John Stuart, *On Liberty*

Odent, Michel, **1984**, *Birth Reborn*, Pantheon

Odent, Michel, **1986**, *Primal Health*, Century Hutchinson

Odent, Michel, **1989**, *Le Bébé est un mammifère*, Fine Line

Padilla, S G, **1935**, 'Further Studies in the Delayed Pecking of Chicks', *Journal of Comparative Psychology*, 20

Piaget, Jean, **1936**, *The Origin of Intelligence in the Child*, first published in English by Routledge and Kegan Paul (1953)

Piaget, Jean, **1951** (first English edition), *Play, Dreams and Imitation in Childhood*, Routledge and Kegan Paul; also William Heinemann (1962)

Richman, Geoffrey, *Fly a Flag for Poplar* (the book of the film), Liberation Films

Roszak, Theodore, **1977**, *Person/Planet*, Victor Gollancz (1979) and Granada Publishing (1981)

Scott, Drusilla, **1985**, *Everyman Revived: the common sense of Michael Polanyi*, The Book Guild

Shinn, Milicent W, **1900**, *The Biography of a Baby*, reprinted by Addison-Wesley (1985)

Shinn, Milicent W, **1909**, *Notes on the Development of a Child*, Berkeley

Stallibrass, Alison, **1974**, *The Self-Respecting Child*, Thames and Hudson; also Pelican Books (1977) and Addison-Wesley (1989)

Thomas, Elizabeth Marshall, **1959**, *The Harmless People*, Alfred A Knopf

Tinbergen, Niko, **1972**, 'The Croonian Lecture: Functional Ethology and the Human Sciences', *Proceedings of the Royal Society*, B182

Tinbergen, Niko, **1976**, 'Tasks for Ethology', *Growing Points in Ethology*, Bateson and Hinde (eds), Cambridge University Press

Tinbergen, Niko and E A, **1983**, *Autistic Children: new hope for a cure*, George Allen and Unwin

Turnbull, Colin, **1961**, *The Forest People*, Jonathan Cape; also Picador (1979)

Turnbull, Colin, **1982**, 'The Ritualisation of Potential Conflict among the Mbuti', *Politics and History in Band Societies*, Leacock, E and Lee, R (eds), Cambridge University Press

White, Robert Winthrop, **1959**, 'Motivation Reconsidered: the concept of competence', *Psychological Review*, Vol. 66, No. 5, reprinted in Hollander, E P and Hunt, R G (eds), *Current Perspectives in Social Psychology* (1963)

White, Robert Winthrop, **1972**, *The Enterprise of Living: a view of personal Growth*, Holt, Rinehardt and Winston

Williams, Roger J, **1967**, *You are Extraordinary*, Pyramid Books (1974)

Index